Medications for the Treatment of Diabetes

R. Keith Campbell, RPh, FASHP, FAPhA,, CDE
John R. White, Jr., PA-C, PharmD

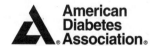

American
Diabetes
Association

Director, Book Publishing	John Fedor
Book Acquisitions	Robert J. Anthony
Editor	Aime M. Ballard
Production Manager	Peggy M. Rote
Composition	Harlowe Typography, Inc.
Text and Cover Design	Wickham & Associates, Inc.
Printer	Transcontinental Printing, Inc.

Printed in Canada

1 3 5 7 9 10 8 6 4 2

The suggestions and information contained in this publication are generally consistent with the *Clinical Practice Recommendations* and other policies of the American Diabetes Association, but they do not represent the policy or position of the Association or any of its boards or committees. Reasonable steps have been taken to ensure the accuracy of the information presented. However, the American Diabetes Association cannot ensure the safety or efficacy of any product or service described in this publication. Individuals are advised to consult a physician or other appropriate health care professional before undertaking any diet or exercise program or taking any medication referred to in this publication. Professionals must use and apply their own professional judgment, experience, and training and should not rely solely on the information contained in this publication before prescribing any diet, exercise, or medication. The American Diabetes Association—its officers, directors, employees, volunteers, and members— assumes no responsibility or liability for personal or other injury, loss, or damage that may result from the suggestions or information in this publication.

∞ The paper in this publication meets the requirements of the ANSI Standard Z39.48-1992 (permanence of paper).

ADA titles may be purchased for business or promotional use or for special sales. For information, please write to: Lee Romano Sequeira, Special Sales & Promotions, at the address below.

American Diabetes Association
1701 North Beauregard Street
Alexandria, Virginia 22311

Library of Congress Cataloging-in-Publication Data
Campbell, R. Keith, 1941-
    Medications for the treatment of diabetes / R. Keith Campbell, John R. White, Jr.
      p. ; cm.
    Includes bibliographical references and index.
    ISBN 1-58040-036-1 (pbk : alk. paper)
    1. Hypoglycemic agents. 2. Diabetes—Chemotherapy. I. White, John R. Jr., 1958-
II. Title.
    [DNLM: 1. Diabetes Mellitus—drug therapy. 2. Antihypertensive Agents— administration & dosage. 3. Drug Interactions. 4. Drug Monitoring. 5. Hypoglycemic Agents—administration & dosage. 6. Insulin—administration & dosage.
WK 815 C189m 2000]
RC661.A1 C25 2000
616.4'62061—dc21   00-029307

Contents

Preface

Diabetes is a fascinating yet devastating disorder that continues to be a major cause of morbidity and mortality in the United States and throughout the world. In the past 10 years, our understanding of hyperglycemia and its causes and consequences has grown dramatically. The more we know, the more we know that there is still much more to know. Our appreciation of the complexity of diabetes and of the efforts that people with diabetes need to undertake each day to try to reach near-normal blood glucose levels is at an all-time high. The basic formula to achieve treatment objectives has been with us for a long time, however. Patients need to be empowered through education and motivation to follow a daily treatment program that includes nutrition, exercise, drug therapy, and self-monitoring. It is important that the patient and the health care provider understand and use each step in the treatment program to control blood glucose levels and slow the development of diabetes complications.

In the past 5 years, the tool chest of medications has grown significantly. We have progressed from insulin and sulfonylureas to new and better medications in these classes and to medications that reduce the liver's release of glucose, that slow the absorption of carbohydrates, and that decrease insulin resistance and increase insulin sensitivity. Medications in many ways are the simplest of all the treatment options. They are more successful in terms of outcomes than nutrition or exercise alone and are the most cost-effective of the treatment alternatives. It is very important to remember, however, that medications are most successful when used in combination with nutrition, exercise, and self-monitoring in an educated, motivated patient.

Medications for the Treatment of Diabetes was written to provide physicians, nurses, dietitians, pharmacists, physician assistants, nurse practitioners, exercise physiologists, psychologists, and motivated patients with an in-depth but easy-to-use summary of the medications used to treat patients with type 1 or type 2 diabetes. The book is written to give an overview of the medications and to provide an individual summary of each class of drugs and its role in the treatment of diabetes. Chapters are included that summarize the two other disease states that are commonly associated with insulin resistance—hypertension and hyper-lipidemia—and the final chapter gives brief descriptions of medications currently being studied that will possibly be approved to treat diabetes or its complications. The authors, editors, contributors, and the American Diabetes Association believe that you will find this book of great value in understanding and using medications to improve the care of your patients with diabetes.

Authors

R. Keith Campbell, RPh, FASHP, FAPhA, CDE
Associate Dean/Professor of Pharmacy Practice
College of Pharmacy, Washington State University

John R. White, Jr., PA-C, PharmD
Associate Professor of Pharmacy Practice
Director, Drug Studies Unit
College of Pharmacy, Washington State University at Spokane

Contributors

Danial E. Baker, PharmD, FASCP, FASHP
Professor of Pharmacy Practice
Director, Drug Information Center
College of Pharmacy, Washington State University at Spokane

Lance K. Campbell, PharmD, MHA
Assistant Professor of Pharmacy Practice
College of Pharmacy, Washington State University

1. Understanding Medications Used to Treat Type 1 Diabetes

INTRODUCTION

Insulin is a hormone produced in the β-cells of pancreatic islets in individuals with normal pancreatic function (1). Stimulation of the pancreas by elevations in blood glucose levels results in the release of insulin from β-cells into the circulation, where it exerts varied effects on body tissues. The glucose-lowering effects of insulin are the result of its ability to stimulate glucose utilization and promote glycogenesis (glycogen storage) in hepatic and skeletal muscle cells, to inhibit glycogenolysis (glucose production) in the liver and skeletal muscle, and to inhibit gluconeogenesis (glucose formation) from amino acids and other non-carbohydrates. Type 1 diabetes is characterized by a deficiency in endogenous insulin secretion, and affected individuals depend on injections of exogenous insulin to survive (2).

Insulin was first isolated and made available for clinical use in the 1920s (3). Over the past two decades, however, therapeutic strategies for diabetes management have changed significantly, and major advances have been made in the way therapy is used in clinical practice (4). The progress in diabetes management can be attributed to several factors, primarily the introduction of self-monitoring of blood glucose (SMBG) into routine practice, the impact of patient self-management and flexibility in lifestyle on contemporary treatment approaches, and clinical evidence that tight glycemic control reduces the risk of long-term diabetes-related complications (5). Since the 1960s, the refinement of split-and-mixed insulin programs, the introduction of SMBG into clinical practice, the development of portable insulin pumps, and the use of intensive insulin therapy and flexible insulin therapy have contributed to the evolution of insulin treatment and diabetes management.

INSULIN SOURCES, PURITY, CONCENTRATION

Insulin preparations can be characterized by their time course of action, degree of purity, concentration, and species of origin. Most insulin used in the U.S. today is human insulin. Biosynthetic human insulin and the human insulin analog lispro are manufactured using recombinant DNA techniques; semisynthetic human insulin preparations are manufactured by chemical conversion of porcine insulin to human insulin. Other insulin preparations available in the U.S. are a mixture of porcine and bovine pancreatic products, although these animal-derived insulins have been or soon will be discontinued.

Both human insulin and lispro insulin produce fewer insulin antibodies, resulting in less insulin allergy than animal insulins; therefore, the time course of human insulin is more predictable (6). Purity of animal-source insulin is expressed as parts per million (ppm) of proinsulin, the primary contaminant after extraction from the pancreas (1). Regardless of origin, all insulin preparations in the U.S. are highly purified, resulting in less lipoatrophy at the injection sites.

In the U.S., insulin preparations are available in concentrations of 100 units or 500 units per cubic centimeter, referred to as U-100 and U-500, respectively (1). Nearly all patients on insulin therapy use U-100 insulin; those requiring large doses may find U-500 insulin useful, although the onset and the duration of action of the higher concentration differ from those of U-100 insulin.

INSULIN PHARMACOLOGY

Insulin preparations are generally classified according to their time course of action: rapid-acting, short-acting, intermediate-acting, and long-acting (Table 1.1) (6). Insulin lispro is a genetically engineered human insulin analog that has a rapid onset of action (15–30 min) after subcutaneous injection. The peak effect of insulin lispro occurs 30–90 min after injection, with an effective duration of action of 3–4 h. In some patients the glucose-lowering effect of insulin lispro may be as long as 6 h. Other rapid-acting insulin analogs, including insulin aspart, are in development. In clinical studies comparing insulin aspart with regular human insulin, the time action profile of insulin aspart more closely resembled physiological postprandial insulin release (7) and improved postprandial glucose control in patients with type 1 diabetes (8).

Short-acting insulin consists of regular (soluble) human insulin, which has the most rapid onset and the shortest duration of action of all the natural insulin preparations (6). Regular human insulin has an onset of action of 30–60 min, and the peak effect occurs 2–3 h after

Table 1.1 Comparative Time Course of Action of Insulin Preparations

Insulin Preparation	Onset (h)	Time to Peak Action (h)	Effective Duration of Action (h)	Maximum Duration (h)
Rapid-Acting				
Lispro (analog)	<0.25	0.5–1.5	3–4	4–6
Short-Acting				
Regular (soluble)	0.5–1	2–3	3–6	6–8
Intermediate-Acting				
NPH (isophane)	2–4	6–10	10–16	14–18
Lente (insulin zinc suspension)	3–4	6–12	12–18	16–20
Long-Acting				
Ultralente (extended insulin zinc suspension)	6–10	10–16	18–20	20–24
Glargine (analog)	2	—	24	24
Combinations				
70/30 (70% NPH/30% regular)	0.5–1	dual	10–16	14–18
50/50 (50% NPH/50% regular)	0.5–1	dual	10–16	14–18

Adapted from Skyler (3).

injection. The effective duration of action of regular human insulin lasts from 3 to 6 h, but in some patients the effect may be evident for up to 8 h. Short-acting mixed bovine/porcine insulin preparations are also available with time courses of action similar to that of short-acting human insulin.

The two intermediate-acting insulins currently available in the U.S. are neutral protamine Hagedorn (NPH), or isophane, insulin and lente insulin (1,6). Human NPH insulin, which uses protamine to extend insulin action, has an onset of action 2–4 h after administration, a peak effect at 6–10 h, and an effective duration of action of 10–16 h. Human lente insulin is formulated in a zinc suspension to extend insulin action. The time course of lente insulin is similar to that of NPH insulin but slightly slower, with an onset of action of 3–4 h, a peak effect at 6–12 h, and an effective duration of action of 12–18 h. Mixed bovine/porcine lente insulin preparations are also available but are soon to be discontinued.

The longest time course of action is provided by human ultralente insulin, which has high zinc levels (1,6). Human ultralente insulin has an onset of action 6–10 h after administration. The peak effect occurs 10–16 h after administration, and the duration of the effect can be expected to be 18–20 h.

Several new long-acting insulin analogs are in development or have recently been given U.S. Food and Drug Administration (FDA) approval. Insulin glargine has peakless and prolonged activity compared with NPH insulin, with a delayed onset of action and a significantly prolonged duration of action of ~23 h ($P < 0.002$) (9). The biological action of insulin glargine is not dependent on the addition of zinc to the formulation. Insulin glargine can provide basal insulin needs without producing the peaks of insulin action observed with lente and ultralente formulations (10,11). If injected twice daily at 12-h intervals, insulin glargine is expected to provide near-constant basal insulin levels during the day and a slight decrease in insulin concentrations in the early morning, closely mimicking physiological insulin requirements. The results of a recent study in patients with type 1 diabetes showed that a regimen of preprandial injections of regular insulin and bedtime injections of insulin glargine for 28 weeks was associated with fewer episodes of all forms of hypoglycemia, including nocturnal hypoglycemia, compared with a regimen of preprandial regular insulin and bedtime NPH (12). Glargine cannot be mixed with other insulins. It is the only long- or intermediate-acting insulin that is clear.

NN304 is another investigational insulin analog with a slower onset of action and a diminished peak effect compared with NPH insulin (13). The slow absorption of NN304 is attributed to its reversible binding with albumin (14). NN304 provides a clear dose response, but its pharmacodynamic effects are only 30% of those observed with NPH insulin, such that equal unit doses of NN304 and NPH insulin cannot be considered equipotent.

Premixed combinations of NPH and regular insulin are available that combine the short onset of action (0.5–1.0 h) of regular insulin with the longer effective duration of action (10–16 h) of NPH insulin (6). These mixtures contain 70% NPH and 30% regular insulin ("70/30") or 50% NPH and 50% regular insulin ("50/50").

Premixed formulations of rapid-acting insulins combined with their protamine-based formulations have been approved by FDA; 25% lispro combined with 75% neutral protamine lispro (NPL) and a 50/50 mixture will be available in mid-2000. When mixed with its neutral protamine preparation (NPL insulin), insulin lispro retained its time action profile (15) and provided improved postprandial glycemic control compared with a 70/30 NPH/regular insulin mixture (16,17). Similarly, pharmacological evaluations of a premixed formulation containing 30% insulin aspart, a rapid-acting insulin, and 70% protamine insulin aspart have indicated that this combination has an earlier onset and a more pronounced peak effect than a 30/70 mixture of human insulin/NPH insulin (18). Premixed insulins simplify the mechanics of insulin administration, especially when used in prefilled pens. This is particularly helpful for infants and elderly patients. Premixed preparations are not recommended for patients on intensive insulin programs because the dose of rapid-acting insulin cannot be adjusted.

Insulin absorption can be affected by many factors and can vary in the same individual by ~25% from day to day (6). There appears to be somewhat less variation in the absorption of rapid- and short-acting insulins and more variation in absorption of longer-acting insulins. Insulin regimens that emphasize shorter-acting insulins therefore have more reproducible effects on blood glucose.

Absorption also varies according to the site of injection (1). Insulin is absorbed most rapidly from the abdomen, followed by the arm, buttocks, and thigh. It is preferable to rotate injection sites within a particular region, rather than between regions, for any particular (e.g., prebreakfast) injection. The choice of injection site can be influenced by the patient's lifestyle and individual insulin program. For example, injection into the thigh, from which absorption is slowest, can provide basal insulin levels for 15 h or more; in contrast, injection into the abdomen may be preferred for preprandial injections, since absorption is most rapid from this site.

Other factors that affect insulin absorption include physical exercise, which accelerates absorption because of increased blood flow; ambient temperature; smoking; and local massage of the injection site.

INSULIN STORAGE, MIXING, AND ADMINISTRATION

The correct equipment and insulin preparation and consistent use of proper technique are crucial to the effective use of insulin (1). Insulin should be stored according to the manufacturer's recommendations. Generally, insulin should be refrigerated at 36–46°F (2–8°C). Unopened products can be stored under refrigeration until the expiration date on the product label. Table 1.2 gives storage times for insulin in different forms. The following are additional storage guidelines (1):

- Patient-prepared, prefilled syringes of single insulin formulations or insulin mixtures should be refrigerated and used within 21–30 days.
- Insulin may be affected by variances in temperature, particularly during car or plane travel.

Table 1.2 Insulin Storage Limits

	Refrigerated	Room Temperature
Unopened vials	Expiration date	1 month
Opened vials	1–2 months*	1 month
Cartridges for pens		
Regular and lispro	Expiration date	1 month
NPH and 70/30	Expiration date	7 days
Disposable pens (Lilly)		
Lispro	Expiration date	14 days
NPH	Expiration date	10 days

*Opened vials lose potency over time, even when refrigerated.

- Insulin should be protected from direct sunlight.
- Vials of insulin should be examined for sediment, cloudiness, discoloration, or clumping or frosting of insulin suspensions before use.

Guidelines for mixing individual insulin products are given in Table 1.3 (1). In general, errors can be reduced by organizing the necessary equipment before the insulin injection. The two insulins to be mixed should be of the same brand. Drawing up lispro or regular insulin before drawing up the intermediate-acting insulin will reduce the risk of contamination and subsequent dose variability. Differences in insulin action may occur if the mixed insulin is injected at varying times after mixing. The commercially available premixed insulins are stabilized and may be preferable for patients unable to mix insulins accurately or reliably.

The traditional equipment used for U-100 insulin administration is a disposable syringe with attached needles (1). A variety of syringe sizes, ranging from 0.25 cc to 1 cc, is available to accommodate the dose of insulin to be injected. Needle length may be 5/16 or 1/2 inch. Several injection devices have been developed as alternatives to the syringe-needle unit, including automatic needle injectors, automatic needle and insulin injectors, pen injectors, and needle-free jet injectors. Insulin pumps, or continuous subcutaneous insulin infusion (CSII) devices, are programmed to deliver a continuous infusion of insulin subcutaneously (see Insulin Pump Therapy below).

For insulin therapy to be effective, a specific routine for insulin injections must be established that includes consistent technique, accurate dosage, and site rotation. Injections are given into the subcutaneous tissue of a fold of skin, with the needle at a 90° angle for most adults or at

Table 1.3 Guidelines for Mixing Insulin and/or Prefilling Syringes

Insulin Preparations to be Mixed	Important Considerations
Lispro with NPH or ultralente	■ Mixture stable in any ratio ■ Administer immediately after mixing
Regular and NPH	■ Mixture stable in any ratio ■ Prefilling is acceptable ■ Patient-prepared syringes stable for at least 1 month if refrigerated
Regular and lente	■ Binding of regular insulin begins immediately and continues for 24 h ■ Activity of regular insulin is blunted ■ Interval between mixing the insulins and administering the injections should be standardized but administer immediately after mixing if possible
Lente and ultralente	■ Mixture stable in any ratio ■ Mixture stable for 18 months ■ Prefilling is acceptable but rarely done
Commercially prepared premixed insulins	■ Prefilling is acceptable
Glargine	■ Cannot be mixed with other insulins

From White et al. (1).

a 45° angle for thin adults or children. Commonly used injection sites include the abdomen, upper arm, thigh, and hip. Factors that influence the choice of injection site include patient preference, presence of scar tissue, amount of subcutaneous fat, and rate of absorption. Injection sites should be rotated to prevent local irritation, and the areas should be examined to detect any redness, bruising, infection, lipoatrophy, or lipohypertrophy.

INSULIN DOSING REGIMENS

Since the primary defect in type 1 diabetes is insulin deficiency, treatment consists of attempting to mimic physiological insulin secretion by the pancreas, i.e., continuous basal release with additional bursts of insulin released in proportion to the demand required by the size and nature of each meal (2). Basal insulin requirements may vary due to physical stress, hormonal changes, illness, physical activity, and level of physical fitness. In the nondiabetic state, insulin is released into the portal circulation. This allows for a "first-pass" effect by the liver before insulin is released into the systemic circulation. This first-pass effect is responsible for regulating hepatic glucose production. Because of these differences, physiological insulin replacement can only be approximated with current insulins.

Designing an insulin regimen is a process of working with the patient to find a regimen that provides adequate coverage and flexibility with respect to meals, physical activity, schedule, other medications, and emotional factors. For most patients with type 1 diabetes, achieving adequate glycemic control and flexibility requires using multidose regimens (3–4 injections per day). In many situations, compromises must be made to achieve the best glycemic control possible with a regimen that the patient is willing to use.

Twice-Daily Regimens

The simplest regimen for treating type 1 diabetes is two insulin injections per day. Twice-daily regimens consist of one dose of intermediate-acting insulin alone or mixed with lispro or regular insulin administered in the morning and another dose before supper (2). Fig. 1.1 depicts the idealized insulin effect of such a twice-daily "split-mixed" insulin regimen, often considered conventional insulin therapy (1). With the morning dose, the rapid-acting (lispro) or short-acting (regular) insulin provides a major effect between breakfast and lunch, and the intermediate-acting (NPH or lente) insulin exerts its major action between breakfast and supper. When administered before supper, the short-acting insulin has its major effect between supper and bedtime, and the intermediate-acting insulin provides its major action overnight to reduce morning glucose levels. Twice-daily dosing results in better blood glucose management if the patient does not eat lunch or eats only a small lunch; if the patient eats a larger lunch, a three-injection regimen may be necessary to control blood glucose.

The timing of administration of the premeal insulin can affect postprandial glucose control. For example, when the premeal blood glucose level is 80–200 mg/dl (4.4–11.1 mmol/l), regular insulin has its optimal

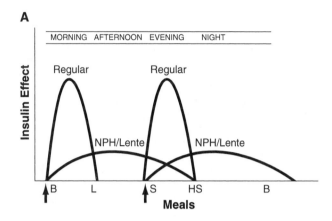

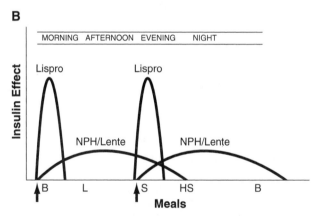

Figure 1.1 Schematic representation of the idealized insulin effect of a twice-daily split-mixed insulin regimen using regular (*A*) or lispro (*B*) as the short-acting insulin. From Skyler (2).

effect when given 30–45 min before the meal. When the premeal glucose is >200 mg/dl (11.1 mmol/l), the meal should be delayed (up to 60 minutes) to allow the regular insulin to take effect. Lispro insulin, because of its more rapid action, is equally effective when taken 0–15 min before or after the meal when the premeal glucose is in the normal range (19). When the premeal glucose is >180 mg/dl (10.0 mmol/l), lispro should be administered 15–30 min before the meal (20).

Flexible

Multiple-component flexible insulin programs attempt to mimic endogenous preprandial insulin levels as well as basal insulin levels overnight and between meals (1–3). Flexible insulin regimens typically involve three daily injections consisting of preprandial injections of a rapid- or short-acting insulin (lispro or regular) before each meal and an injection of a long-acting insulin (ultralente) at night (Fig. 1.2). The preprandial component of flexible insulin therapy adjusts the dose to be appropriate to the size of the meal and allows for flexibility in meal timing (6).

Alternatively, an injection of an intermediate-acting insulin (NPH or lente) in the morning and again at bedtime may be used instead of the single injection of a long-acting insulin (Fig. 1.3). The rationale for this approach is the effect of the bedtime intermediate-acting insulin to reduce the risk of nocturnal hypoglycemia and coverage for early morning hyperglycemia with the release of growth hormone (1).

USE OF INSULIN IN SPECIAL SITUATIONS/POPULATIONS

Diabetic Ketoacidosis

Diabetic ketoacidosis (DKA) is a serious, acute metabolic complication of diabetes that occurs in 2–5% of patients with type 1 diabetes each year, with a mortality rate of up to 10%, primarily from sepsis or pulmonary or cardiovascular complications (21–24). The diagnostic triad for DKA consists of hyperglycemia, high levels of ketone bodies, and metabolic acidosis, each of which is usually associated with other diseases or metabolic conditions. Any known diabetic patient with nausea or vomiting, abdominal pain, central nervous system depression, shortness of breath, fever, localized signs of infection, or unexplained hyperglycemia (>250 mg/dl [13.9 mmol/l]) is a candidate for DKA.

The essential components of treatment in adults and children are potassium repletion, fluid replacement, and insulin administration (21,22). Potassium replacement is essential to prevent death from cardiac arrhythmia or respiratory arrest. Adequate rehydration is important to restore and maintain circulating volume and to enhance kidney function to excrete glucose and reduce hyperglycemia. Rehydration alone, however, is inadequate in reducing hyperglycemia in the presence of absolute or relative insulin deficiency in DKA. Therefore, insulin must be administered to reduce plasma glucose levels and correct acidosis.

In adults, a short-acting (regular) rather than intermediate-acting (NPH or lente) insulin should be used for treatment of DKA (Table 1.4)

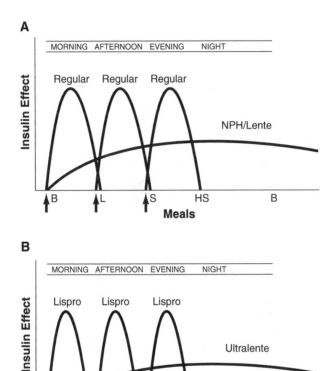

Figure 1.2 Schematic representation of the idealized insulin effect with a three-daily-injection regimen using preprandial regular (*A*) or lispro (*B*) as the short-acting insulin and a long-acting insulin. From Skyler (2).

(21,25). The insulin should be administered as a continuous intravenous infusion in a starting dose of 10 U i.v. push followed by 0.1 U/kg/h via pump. An initial intravenous bolus of 10 U i.v. will provide an immediate therapeutic level of insulin while the other components of the treatment regimen are being prepared. Plasma glucose levels should decrease at a rate of 75 mg/dl/h (4.2 mmol/l/h) in response to insulin. A lack of response in 4 h is indicative of an unusual degree of insulin resistance and requires an increase in the intravenous dose of short-acting insulin to

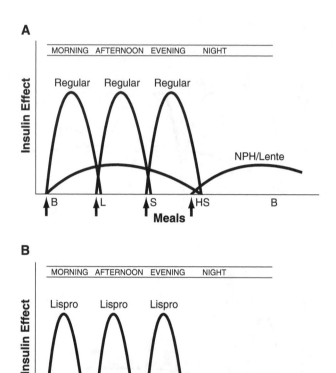

Figure 1.3 Schematic representation of the idealized insulin effect with a four-daily-injection regimen using preprandial regular (*A*) or lispro (*B*) as the short-acting insulin and an intermediate-acting insulin in the morning and at bedtime

20–100 U/h depending on the degree of hyperglycemia. The dose can be doubled further every 2 h until plasma glucose levels decline. Within 4–8 h of the start of insulin therapy, its effectiveness should be reflected in the return of plasma bicarbonate and anion gap to normal levels. When plasma glucose levels have reached 250 mg/dl (13.9 mmol/l), glucose should be added to the replacement fluids to allow for the continued administration of insulin. This allows for complete normalization of

Table 1.4 Administration of Short-Acting Insulin in the Treatment of Diabetic Ketoacidosis in Adults

Intravenous Administration
- 10 U short-acting (regular) insulin by intravenous bolus followed by continuous intravenous infusion at 0.1 U/kg/h
- If no response by 4 h, increase dose 2- to 10-fold
- Decrease dose to 1–2 U/h when acidosis is corrected
- Administer 4–10 U short-acting insulin subcutaneously before discontinuing infusion

Intramuscular Administration*
- 0.5 U/kg for first hour of therapy
- 0.1 U/kg each hour subsequently, until blood glucose levels decline to 250 mg/dl (13.9 mmol/l)
- 0.1 U/kg every 2 h thereafter as necessary to maintain blood glucose levels of 200–250 mg/dl (11.1–13.9 mmol/l)

*Only if intravenous infusion cannot be performed. Adapted from Genuth (21) and Skyler (25).

ketone levels and maintenance of blood glucose levels at 150–250 mg/dl (8.3–13.9 mmol/l) with minimal risk of hypoglycemia. Once the patient is capable of oral intake, 4–10 U of short-acting insulin should be administered subcutaneously at least 30 min before discontinuation of the intravenous infusion.

DKA in children represents a true pediatric medical emergency because of the risk of cerebral edema and associated morbidity and mortality (26). The treatment approach is similar to that in adults, i.e., correction of potassium depletion and of dehydration and administration of insulin for complete correction of ketosis. However, pediatric patients need to be monitored diligently for signs and symptoms of intracerebral crisis during treatment.

Pregnant Women

Insulin therapy is used to maintain glycemic control during pregnancy in women with type 1 diabetes, as well as in many pregnant women with either type 2 or gestational diabetes (27). Women with diabetes are at increased risk of giving birth to infants with congenital abnormalities (27). Therefore, the goal of therapy is to normalize blood glucose before conception and maintain glycemic control during critical periods of fetal development. A flexible insulin regimen can be developed based on the results of SMBG, the meal plan, and the exercise regimen (Table 1.5) (25). One regimen involves three daily injections: the patient's usual morning dose of intermediate- and short-acting insulins, a suppertime injection of short-acting insulin, and a bedtime injection of intermediate-acting insulin. The greatest flexibility is provided by a four-injection regimen that consists of mixed intermediate- and short-acting insulins at breakfast, short-acting insulin at lunch and supper, and intermediate- or long-acting insulin at bedtime. Insulin can also be administered by continuous subcutaneous infusion via pump.

Infants and Children

Type 1 diabetes affects an estimated 130,000 children under 20 years of age in the U.S., and approximately 13,000 new cases are diagnosed each year (28). The goals of diabetes management in these children are to achieve normal physical and emotional growth, to reduce the symptoms that result from hypoglycemia or hyperglycemia, and to lessen the risk of long-term complications.

Insulin therapy for pediatric type 1 diabetes can be a challenge. It is often difficult to simulate normal physiological fluctuations in plasma insulin levels because of the severe insulin deficit in children and because of psychosocial considerations of acceptability and compliance (29). The insulin regimen needs to be tailored for the individual child and adjusted as the child grows and develops. The dose of insulin will increase steadily as weight and caloric intake increase with age, as any residual endogenous insulin secretion declines and the child or adolescent becomes completely insulin deficient (usually 2–3 years after diagnosis), and as the hormonal and physiological changes of puberty induce a state of relative insulin resistance (29). Adolescents with well-controlled glycemia

---

Table 1.5 Proposed Insulin Regimen for Pregnant Women with Diabetes

Four Injections a Day
▪ Short-acting insulin at breakfast
▪ Short-acting insulin at lunch
▪ Short-acting insulin at dinner
▪ Intermediate- or long- (ultralente) acting insulin at bedtime

Adapted from Skyler (25) and Reece and Homko (27).

may require daily insulin doses between 1.5 and 3 U/kg. Day-to-day adjustments to the prebreakfast and predinner insulins may be needed to accommodate daily fluctuations in preprandial glucose levels.

Most children will accept a twice-daily injection regimen consisting of a mixture of intermediate-acting (NPH or lente) and short-acting (regular or lispro) insulins in a total dose of (1.0–1.5 U/kg/day (Table 1.6) (29). The first daily dose is administered before breakfast and contains two-thirds of the total dose in a ratio of 2:1 of intermediate- to short-acting insulin. The remaining one-third of the total dose is given as a second injection before supper. During the early phases of treatment, the ratio of intermediate- to short-acting insulins may need to be adjusted for adequate control of prebreakfast and predinner glucose levels, and preprandial rapid-acting insulin can be added, if needed.

With the twice-daily regimen, the peak effect of the predinner intermediate-acting insulin often coincides with the nocturnal minimal insulin requirement and diminishes as basal insulin requirements increase in early morning (29). This and other difficulties of the two-

Table 1.6 Proposed Insulin Regimen for Children with Type 1 Diabetes

Twice-Daily Regimen	Intensified Insulin Therapy
■ Total daily dose of ~1.0–1.5 U/kg administered in two divided doses	■ More aggressive regimen containing long-, intermediate-, and short-acting insulins
■ Two-thirds of total daily dose administered as 2:1 ratio of intermediate- and short-acting insulins before breakfast	■ Three-times-daily regimen: mixed intermediate- and short-acting insulins at breakfast, short-acting insulin at dinner, and intermediate-acting insulin at bedtime; long-acting may be substituted for morning NPH to give better coverage in the afternoon
■ Remaining one-third administered before dinner	
■ Ratio of intermediate-acting to short-acting insulin can be adjusted for acceptable prebreakfast and predinner glucose levels	■ Substitute long-acting insulin for basal insulin and use short-acting insulin before each meal
■ Preprandial doses of rapid-acting insulin can be added if needed.	

Adapted from Tamborlane et al. (29).

injection regimen may be overcome by more intensive insulin therapy using long-acting (ultralente) insulin alone or in combination with intermediate-acting (NPH or lente) insulin, short-acting (regular or lispro) insulin, or both. Alternatively, a three-injection regimen, consisting of mixed intermediate- and short-acting insulins at breakfast, short-acting insulin at supper, and intermediate-acting insulin at bedtime (Table 1.6) may alleviate this problem. In addition, long-acting insulin may be substituted for the morning NPH to compensate for late-afternoon snacks and to maintain normal predinner glucose levels. CSII with a portable pump also more closely simulates normal physiological insulin profiles and provides an alternative to multiple daily injections for highly motivated and responsible patients. CSII is being used with greater frequency in children and in type 2 patients who use insulin.

The Diabetes Control and Complications Trial demonstrated that intensive insulin therapy delayed the onset and progression of diabetes-related retinopathy and nephropathy in a subset of patients aged 13–18 years (29). Therefore, it appears that the benefits of intensified insulin treatment in adolescents may outweigh the risks of hypoglycemia that can accompany intensive treatment.

Parenteral Nutrition

Acute hyperglycemia can occur in diabetic and nondiabetic patients alike who are receiving enteral or parenteral nutrition (30). Hundreds of formulas are available for tube feeding, but one formula low in carbohydrates (38%) is used in patients with diabetes who require nutritional support. These patients should be given regular insulin for their basal and formula-related needs. Enteral nutrition and the insulin infusion are started simultaneously. The dose of insulin for basal need is calculated according to the patient's stress level and whether glucocorticoid therapy is needed, and it ranges from 0.3 U to a maximum of 1 U/kg body weight (Table 1.7). To meet carbohydrate-related needs, the starting dose of regular insulin is 1 U for every 10 g carbohydrate in the enteral nutrition formula. Blood glucose levels should be monitored every 4 h, and additional units of regular insulin can be administered subcutaneously if levels are elevated (Table 1.7). For subsequent enteral feedings, the ratio of insulin units to grams of carbohydrate is adjusted based on current blood glucose levels (Table 1.7).

Similarly, hyperglycemia can occur after administration of peripheral parenteral solutions containing 10% dextrose or central parenteral solutions containing 20% dextrose (30). The same basal insulin requirements and insulin dose adjustments apply to parenteral nutrition for patients with type 1 diabetes (Table 1.7). Blood glucose levels should be monitored every 4 h for 2 days and twice daily thereafter if levels remain

Table 1.7 Insulin Treatment for Patients with Type 1 Diabetes on Enteral or Parenteral Nutrition Therapy

	Basal Insulin Need: Regular Insulin	If glucose level during enteral therapy is	Carbohydrate- or Dextrose-Related Need (1 U/10 g carbohydrate)		
			Give additional regular insulin subcutaneously	If current blood glucose level is	Adjust subsequent insulin ratio
Stress Level					
Mild	0.3 U/kg	<180 mg/dl (10 mmol/l)	None	<80 mg/dl (4.4 mmol/l)	0.5 U/10 g carbohydrate or dextrose
Moderate	0.5 U/kg	181–240 mg/dl (10.1–13.3 mmol/l)	6 U	81–180 mg/dl (4.5–10 mmol/l)	1 U/10 g carbohydrate or dextrose
Severe	1.0 U/kg	241–300 mg/dl (13.4–16.7 mmol/l)	8 U	>181 mg/dl (10 mmol/l)	1.5 U/10 g carbohydrate or dextrose
Steroid Therapy	1.0 U/kg	>301 mg/dl (16.7 mmol/l)	10 U		

From Jovanovic-Peterson and Peterson (30).

normal. The amount of additional insulin needed is based on the amount of dextrose in the parenteral solution, starting with a dose of 1 U of regular insulin for every 10 g dextrose; and the ratio of insulin units to dextrose amount for subsequent parenteral nutrition is adjusted based on current blood glucose levels (Table 1.7).

Insulin Pump Therapy

Continuous subcutaneous insulin infusion (CSII), or insulin pump therapy, is an adjustable method of subcutaneous insulin administration that can vastly improve glycemic control and reduce the risk of hypoglycemia (31,32). For patients with type 2 diabetes highly motivated to achieve glycemic control, CSII is an alternative to multiple daily injections that fail to meet glycemic goals. CSII systems are small, accurate, reliable, and easy to use. They consist of a pump and an infusion set small enough to be carried in a pocket, worn on a belt, or hidden under clothing.

Insulin therapy by CSII approximates the normal physiological fluctuations in plasma insulin more closely than multiple injections by maintaining a basal rate of rapid-acting insulin that consists of 40–60% of the total daily dose and by delivering preprandial bolus doses (33). Basal insulin delivery usually ranges from 0.4 to 2.0 U/h, and the pump can be programmed to deliver different basal rates over a 24-h period. In addition, bolus doses can be programmed to allow for some flexibility in meal schedules with minimal risk of hypoglycemia (31,32).

The glucose-lowering effects of CSII are highly predictable because insulin is delivered at a precise rate and programmed according to the patient's need (31,32). Preprandial bolus doses are calculated according to the amount and carbohydrate content of the meal, usually 1 U of insulin for each 10–15 g carbohydrate, or as a percentage of the total daily dose (33). In general, the blood glucose target is 80–140 mg/dl (4.4–7.8 mmol/l) for the average of capillary blood glucose values taken before each meal and at bedtime. Furthermore, the patient can be taught to adjust the basal rate and bolus doses for exercise, illness, and between-meal hyperglycemia. Compared with regular insulin, the rapid-acting insulin lispro can provide improved postprandial glucose reduction and fluctuations with no increased risk of hypoglycemic episodes (33,34).

Some of the risks of insulin pump therapy include skin infections, which can be avoided or resolved with meticulous skin care; unexplained hyperglycemia, which usually results from an interruption in insulin delivery; and hypoglycemia, which can be minimized by frequent monitoring of blood glucose levels (33). According to pump manufacturer surveys, over 80% of pump users are now using lispro insulin.

ROLE OF GLUCAGON IN TYPE 1 DIABETES

Glucagon is a hormone used to treat symptomatic hypoglycemia, particularly when intravenous glucose is not readily available or an intravenous line cannot be established (35–37). It acts by activating enzymes in hepatic cells that increase glycogenolysis and gluconeogenesis, thereby increasing hepatic glucose production. Immediate clinical improvement is necessary to avoid the risk of neurological damage caused by severe hypoglycemia. However, the action of glucagon may be inadequate if hepatic stores of glycogen are depleted. Recurrent hypoglycemia can be prevented if the patient is given glucose or is urged to eat after the initial response to glucagon. Nausea and vomiting may occur after administration of glucagon.

A 1- to 2-mg dose of glucagon administered intramuscularly or subcutaneously can increase blood glucose levels within minutes, and the effect is sustained for ~30 min (36). Studies of patients requiring emergency medical treatment for hypoglycemia have shown that although the time from diagnosis of severe hypoglycemia to full neurological orientation is longer after intramuscular glucagon than after intravenous glucose ($P < 0.05$), glucagon is a safe and reliable alternative to intravenous glucose (37,38).

Avoiding severe hypoglycemia is particularly important in children and adolescents with type 1 diabetes (39). Although most episodes of hypoglycemia can be treated with rapidly absorbed glucose or a form of rapidly absorbed carbohydrate (e.g., table sugar or fruit juice), a glucagon emergency kit should be available in the home and family members should be instructed in its use for treatment of severe hypoglycemia. The kit contains a syringe filled with diluent and a vial of lyophilized hormone. After subcutaneous administration, the child's blood glucose level will increase in 5–15 min. Oral glucose should be provided within 15–20 min of the injection to avoid further hypoglycemia. Some children may continue to be symptomatic for an extended period of time despite an apparently normal blood glucose level. As in adults, glucagon administration may cause nausea and vomiting in children.

REFERENCES

1. White JR Jr, Campbell RK, Yarborough PC: Pharmacologic therapies. In *A Core Curriculum for Diabetes Education.* Funnell MM, Hunt C, Kulkarni K, Rubin RR, Yarborough PC, Eds. Chicago, American Association of Diabetes Educators, 1998, pp. 297–358

2. Skyler JS (Ed.): Routine management: tools. In *Medical Management of Type 1 Diabetes*. 3rd ed. Alexandria, VA, American Diabetes Association, 1998, pp. 55–83

3. Skyler JS: Insulin treatment. In *Therapy for Diabetes Mellitus and Related Disorders*. 3rd ed. Lebovitz HE, Ed. Alexandria, VA, American Diabetes Association, 1998, pp. 186–203

4. Skyler JS: Tactics for type 1 diabetes. *Endocrinol Metab Clin North Am* 26:647–657, 1997

5. The Diabetes Control and Complications Trial Research Group: The effect of intensive treatment of diabetes on the development and progression of long-term complications in insulin-dependent diabetes mellitus. *N Engl J Med* 329:977–986, 1993

6. Farkas-Hirsch R (Ed.): Multiple-component insulin regimens. In *Intensive Diabetes Management*. 2nd ed. Alexandria, VA, American Diabetes Association, 1998, pp. 73–98

7. Home PD, Barriocanal L, Lindholm A: Comparative pharmacokinetics and pharmacodynamics of the novel rapid-acting insulin analogue, insulin aspart, in healthy volunteers. *Eur J Clin Pharmacol* 55:199–203, 1999

8. Home PD, Lindholm A, Hylleberg B, Round P: Improved glycemic control with insulin aspart: a multicenter randomized double-blind crossover trial in type 1 diabetic patients: UK Insulin Aspart Study Group. *Diabetes Care* 21:1904–1909, 1998

9. Lepore M, Kurzhals R, Pampanelli S, Fanelli CG, Bolli GB: Pharmacokinetics and dynamics of s.c. injection of the long-acting insulin glargine (HOE1) in T1DM (Abstract). *Diabetes* 48 (Suppl. 1):A97, 1999

10. Hirsch IB: Intensive treatment of type 1 diabetes. *Med Clin North Am* 82:689–719, 1998

11. Coates PA, Mukherjee S, Luzio S, Srodzinski KA, Kurzhals R, Roskamp R, Owens DR: Pharmacokinetics of a "long-acting" human insulin analogue (HOE901) in healthy subjects (Abstract). *Diabetes* 44 (Suppl. 1):130A, 1995

12. Ratner RE, Hirsch IB, Mecca TE, Wilson CA: Efficacy and safety of insulin glargine in subjects with type 1 diabetes: a 28-week randomized, NPH insulin-controlled trial (Abstract). *Diabetes* 48 (Suppl. 1):A120, 1999

13. Heinemann L, Sinha K, Weyer C, Loftager M, Hirschberger S, Heise T: Time-action profile of the soluble, fatty acid acylated, long-acting insulin analogue NN304. *Diabetic Med* 16:332–338, 1999

14. Brunner GA, Sendlhofer G, Wutte A, Ellmerer M, Soegaard B, Seibenhofer A, Hirschberger S, Krejs GT, Pieber TR: Pharmacokinetic and pharmacodynamic properties of insulin analog NN304 in comparison to NPH insulin in humans. *Diabetes* 48 (Suppl. 1):A102, 1999

15. Heise T, Weyer C, Serwas A, Heinrichs S, Osinga J, Roach P, Woodworth J, Gudat U, Heineman L: Time-action profiles of novel premixed preparations of insulin lispro and NPL insulin. *Diabetes Care* 21:800–803, 1998

16. Roach P, Abora V, Yun L, the Humalog Mix25 Study Group: Improved postprandial glycemic control during treatment with Humalog Mix25, a novel protamine-based insulin lispro formulation. *Diabetes Care* 22:1258–1261, 1999

17. Roach P, Trautmann M, Arora V, Sun B, Anderson JH Jr, the Mix50 Study Group: Improved postprandial blood glucose control and reduced nocturnal hypoglycemia during treatment with two novel insulin lispro-protamine formulations, Insulin Lispro Mix25 and Insulin Lispro Mix50. *Clin Ther* 21:523–533, 1999

18. Weyer C, Heise T, Heinemann L: Insulin aspart in a 30/70 premixed formulation: pharmacodynamic properties of a rapid-acting insulin analog in stable mixture. *Diabetes Care* 20:1612–1614, 1997

19. Schernthaner G, Equiluz-Bruck S, Wein W, Bates PC, Sandholzer K, Birkett MA: Postprandial insulin lispro: a new therapeutic option for type 1 diabetic patients. *Diabetes Care* 21:570–573, 1998

20. Rassam AG, Burge MR, Zeise TM, Schade DS: Optimal administration of lispro insulin in hyperglycemic type 1 diabetes. *Diabetes Care* 22:133–136, 1999.

21. Genuth S: Diabetic ketoacidosis and hyperosmolar hyperglycemic nonketotic syndrome in adults. In *Therapy for Diabetes Mellitus and Related Disorders*. 3rd ed. Lebovitz HE, Ed. Alexandria, VA, American Diabetes Association, 1998, pp. 83–96

22. Kitabchi AE, Wall BM: Diabetic ketoacidosis. *Med Clin North Am* 79:9–37, 1995

23. Brink SJ: Diabetic ketoacidosis. *Acta Pediatr Suppl* 427:14–24, 1999

24. Lebovitz HE: Diabetic ketoacidosis. *Lancet* 345:767–772, 1995

25. Skyler JS (Ed.): Special problems. In *Medical Management of Type 1 Diabetes*. 3rd ed. Alexandria, VA, American Diabetes Association, 1998, pp. 122–132

26. Sperling MA: Diabetic ketoacidosis in children. In *Therapy for Diabetes Mellitus and Related Disorders*. 3rd ed. Lebovitz HE, Ed. Alexandria, VA, American Diabetes Association, 1998, pp. 51–60

27. Reece EA, Homko C: Management of pregnant women with diabetes. In *Therapy for Diabetes Mellitus and Related Disorders.* 3rd ed. Lebovitz HE, Ed. Alexandria, VA, American Diabetes Association, 1998, pp. 27–35

28. Kaufman FR: Diabetes in children and adolescents: areas of controversy. *Med Clin North Am* 82:721–737, 1998

29. Tamborlane WV, Gatcomb PM, Savoye M, Ahern J: Type 1 diabetes in children. In *Therapy for Diabetes Mellitus and Related Disorders.* 3rd ed. Lebovitz HE, Ed. Alexandria, VA, American Diabetes Association, 1998, pp. 61–69

30. Jovanovic-Peterson L, Peterson CM: Prescribing insulin for patients on enteral or parenteral nutritional therapy. *Diabetes Professional*, Spring 1991, pp. 15–18

31. Mecklenburg RS: Insulin-pump therapy. In *Therapy for Diabetes Mellitus and Related Disorders.* 3rd ed. Lebovitz HE, Ed. Alexandria, VA, American Diabetes Association, 1998, pp. 204–210

32. Leslie CA: New insulin replacement technologies: overcoming barriers to tight glycemic control. *Cleve Clin J Med* 66:293–302, 1999

33. Farkas-Hirsch R (Ed.): Insulin infusion pump therapy. In *Intensive Diabetes Management.* 2nd ed. Alexandria, VA, American Diabetes Association, 1998, pp. 99–117

34. Bolvin S, Tauber JP, Guerci B, Hanaire H, Lassmann-Vague V, Renard E, Boullu S, Blin P, Augendre-Ferrante B, Pinget M: Improvement in diabetes control with the lispro analog used in external pumps (Abstract). *Horm Metab Res* 30:A8, 1998

35. Kayne DM, Holvey SM: Drugs and hormones that increase blood glucose levels. In *Therapy for Diabetes Mellitus and Related Disorders.* 3rd ed. Lebovitz HE, Ed. Alexandria, VA, American Diabetes Association, 1998, pp. 260–265

36. Kahn CR, Shechter Y: Insulin, oral hypoglycemic agents, and the pharmacology of the endocrine pancreas. In *Goodman and Gilman's The Pharmacological Basis of Therapeutics.* 8th ed. Goodman AG, Rall TW, Nies AS, Taylor P, Eds. New York, McGraw-Hill, 1990, pp. 1463–1495

37. Howell MA, Guly HR: A comparison of glucagon and glucose in prehospital hypoglycaemia. *J Accid Emerg Med* 14:30–32, 1997

38. Carstens S, Sprehn M: Prehospital treatment of severe hypoglycaemia: a comparison of intramuscular glucagon and intravenous glucose. *Prehospital Disaster Med* 13:44–50, 1998

39. Daneman D, Perlman K: Diabetes mellitus in childhood and adolescence. In *Conn's Current Therapy 1999.* Rakel RE, Ed. Philadelphia, Saunders, 1999, pp. 548–555

2. Overview of Medications Used to Treat Type 2 Diabetes

The options available to clinicians in the U.S. for the management of hyperglycemia secondary to type 2 diabetes have changed dramatically in the past decade. Currently there are six categories of medications that may be used in the management of diabetes, including insulins, sulfonylureas, thiazolidinediones, meglitinides, biguanides, and α-glucosidase inhibitors. The efficacy of various permutations of double and triple combination therapies using these medications continues to be evaluated. The selection of the best medication or combinations of medications for the management of hyperglycemia in patients with type 2 diabetes, while based in science, remains to a large degree in the realm of "art." Although in some situations the choice of medication is relatively simple, in the majority of situations the decision-making process is complex and does not necessarily lead to a clear-cut choice. Hopefully, as more is learned about the natural history of diabetes and the pharmacology of the medications used to manage it, the rationale behind medication choice will become more straightforward.

Several factors should be considered when choosing a medication, including degree of glycemic lowering needed to get the patient into target goal ranges, ease of compliance, effect of the medication on lipid profiles, contraindications and side effects, and level of adherence of the patient to the regimen. This chapter will briefly review the use of the above-mentioned categories of medications and will include a discussion of mechanisms of action, efficacy of monotherapy and combination therapy, effects of the medications on lipid profiles, common side effects, contraindications for use of the medications, and patient adherence to the regimens.

SECRETAGOGUES

Two categories of medications, the sulfonylureas and the meglitinides fall into the category known as secretagogues.

Sulfonylureas

Sulfonylureas have been widely used in the management of type 2 diabetes since their introduction in the late 1950s (1). In the past, it was estimated that 40% of all type 2 diabetes patients were treated with sulfonylureas. However, since the introduction of newer oral agents, this number has probably been reduced (1). The sulfonylureas exhibit both pancreatic and extrapancreatic effects and are useful only in patients with viable β-cells (2,3). The primary effect of the sulfonylureas is due to direct stimulation of insulin release (2). In vivo studies of sulfonylureas show that they sensitize β-cells to glucose, increasing insulin secretion indirectly. Therefore, under the influence of sulfonylureas, more insulin is secreted at all glucose levels than would be expected in the absence of sulfonylureas (2). Sulfonylureas may also affect glucose metabolism via several extrapancreatic mechanisms, such as increasing insulin's effect by a postreceptor action, decreasing hepatic insulin extraction, and increasing insulin receptor number and receptor binding affinity; however, the relative clinical relevance of each of these mechanisms of action is still subject to research and debate (2).

Meglitinides

Repaglinide was the first meglitinide compound to be granted Food and Drug Administration (FDA) approval. It is sometimes referred to as a benzoic acid derivative (1). Repaglinide (Prandin) is a nonsulfonylurea insulinotropic agent whose biochemical mechanism of action, closure of ATP-sensitive potassium channels in β-cells, is similar to that of sulfonylureas (4). Closure of ATP-sensitive potassium channels causes an influx of calcium by way of voltage-dependent calcium channels (5). Insulin release is stimulated after intercellular calcium concentrations reach a threshold. Therefore, similar to sulfonylureas, repaglinide reduces blood glucose levels by stimulating insulin release from the pancreas (6).

As with the sulfonylureas, the effectiveness of this compound is dependent on functioning β-cells. It should be noted, however, that repaglinide is structurally unrelated to the sulfonylureas and that in contrast to most sulfonylureas, repaglinide is rapidly absorbed, with maximum concentrations (C_{max}) occurring within 1 h (t_{max}) and is rapidly eliminated ($t_{1/2} < 1$ h) (6). The pharmacodynamic effects of repaglinide roughly parallel its pharmacokinetic profile; thus, this drug is relatively rapid and short acting and is most effective when given before meals (7).

Insulin

Insulin has been used widely for monotherapy since its introduction in 1922 and has been used in combination with oral agents since the late 1950s (1). It has recently been estimated that about one-third of all patients with type 2 diabetes are managed with insulin therapy alone and another 15% with insulin in combination with an oral agent (1).

Insulin binds to the β-subunit of the insulin receptor, activating tyrosine kinase activity of the β-subunit. Activation of tyrosine kinase initiates a cascade of reactions resulting in several physiological events, including inhibition of hepatic glucose production, stimulation of hepatic glucose uptake, stimulation of glucose uptake by muscle, and mild stimulation of glucose uptake by adipose tissue (1). Insulin therapy has been associated with as much as a 44% reduction in hepatic glucose production and between a 17% and 80% increase in peripheral glucose uptake (8).

Biguanides

The biguanide metformin (Glucophage) was first introduced in 1959 as an antihyperglycemic agent for use in patients with type 2 diabetes but was not approved for use in the U.S. until the 1990s (9). Metformin causes several metabolic effects, including changes in lipoprotein and carbohydrate metabolism (8). The effects of this compound on carbohydrate metabolism occur primarily at the level of the liver, inhibiting hepatic glucose production (10). Metformin has no direct effect on β-cell function (11).

α-Glucosidase Inhibitors

Two drugs in the α-glucosidase inhibitor category have been approved for use in the U.S.: acarbose and miglitol. These drugs exhibit mild antihyperglycemic activity. They may be used as monotherapy in newly onset or mild type 2 diabetes and are also useful in combination with insulin or other oral agents in more severe type 2 diabetes.

The primary mechanism of action of α-glucosidase inhibitors is competitive inhibition of the α-glucosidase enzymes in the brush border of the small intestine (12). Additionally, they may inhibit pancreatic α-analase, the enzyme responsible for the hydrolysis of complex starches to oligosaccharides in the lumen of the small intestine. α-glucosidase enzymes are responsible for the breakdown of oligosaccharides, trisaccharides, and disaccharides in the brush border of the small intestine.

These enzymes include maltase, isomaltase, glucoamylase, and sucrase (1). Inhibition of these enzyme systems effectively reduces the rate of absorption of carbohydrates without altering the absolute absorption. The result is reduced postprandial glucose levels. There is a modest effect on fasting glucose.

Thiazolidinediones

The thiazolidinediones are the newest category of medications used in the management of type 2 diabetes. Currently two thiazolidinediones are available for use in the U.S.: pioglitazone and rosiglitazone. A third, troglitazone, was removed from the market in March 2000 because of liver toxicity. These medications appear to work by affecting insulin action without affecting insulin secretion. They are sometimes referred to as insulin sensitizers. Although several mechanisms of action may contribute to their antihyperglycemic properties, it is known that these compounds stimulate receptors on the nuclear surface, PPARγ (peroxisome-proliferator-activated receptor gamma). Therefore, the thiazolidinediones are also referred to as PPAR activators. Stimulation of PPARγ leads to increased glucose uptake by mechanisms that are still unclear. Additionally, these compounds have mild to moderate effects on lipid metabolism (13).

Glycemic Reduction

The level of glycemic reduction afforded by any medication or combination of medications will depend on several factors, including concomitant lifestyle changes, baseline glycemic control, patient compliance, and other medications included in the patient's regimen. These compounding factors make comparisons between studies dubious at best. However, very few head-to-head trials have been carried out comparing the glycemic reduction of one medication to the glycemic reduction of another. To avoid possible bias, package inserts will be used to provide the following data whenever possible. Additional information concerning baseline glycemic control and any other compounding factors will be provided as well. The reader should note that this section is not intended to be a direct comparison of various medications. It is simply a review of the more significant data available. It may, however, be helpful in assisting the practitioner to choose a particular medication or combination of medications.

Sulfonylureas have been associated with a reduction in fasting plasma glucose of between 50 and 70 mg/dl (2.8 and 3.9 mmol/l) and HbA$_{1c}$ reductions of between 1 and 2% (1,11). Several factors have been shown to be predictive of the response to sulfonylureas, including patient age >40 years and actual weight between 110 and 160% of ideal body weight, duration of diabetes <5 years, no prior treatment with insulin or control with <40 U/day, fasting plasma glucose <200 mg/dl (11.1 mmol/l), good β-cell function as evidenced by a high fasting C-peptide level, and absence of islet cell or glutamic acid decarboxylase antibodies (1,11).

Sulfonylurea/insulin combination therapy has been reported to cause an average reduction in fasting plasma glucose levels of between 41 and 43 mg/dl (2.39 mmol/l) when compared with sulfonylurea monotherapy and with meta-analysis. HbA$_{1c}$ levels were reduced by between 0.8 and 1.1% from monotherapeutic baseline in these reviews. Additionally, the average insulin dose reduction was 24% (14,15). Repaglinide has been associated with reductions in HbA$_{1c}$ and fasting plasma glucose levels similar to those achieved with sulfonylurea therapy (1,11).

The ability of insulin therapy to lower blood glucose levels in patients with type 2 diabetes is governed by dose regimen, level of insulin resistance, and probably several other factors. Insulin is effective in reducing blood glucose levels when used as monotherapy and when used in combination with sulfonylureas, metformin, thiazolidinediones, or α-glucosidase inhibitors. The degree of glycemic reduction in patients treated with insulin is dose related. Studies have demonstrated a reduction in fasting plasma glucose of as much as 190 mg/dl (10.5 mmol/l) from baseline with insulin monotherapy (16).

Metformin monotherapy has been associated with a reduction in fasting plasma glucose of 53 mg/dl (2.9 mmol/l) compared with baseline, a postprandial glycemic reduction of 83 mg/dl (4.6 mmol/l) on average versus placebo (baseline not reported), and an HbA$_{1c}$ reduction of 1.4% compared with baseline (17). Acarbose monotherapy given at a dose of 100 mg tid was associated with a reduction in HbA$_{1c}$ levels of 0.77% (6). Before troglitazone was removed from the market, it was approved for combination therapy but not monotherapy (18).

Pioglitazone monotherapy in previously drug-naïve patients was associated with a 2.6% reduction in HbA$_{1c}$ and an 80 mg/dl (4.4 mmol/l) reduction in fasting blood glucose when compared with placebo (19). When given to previously treated patients at a dose of 45 mg/day, pioglitazone resulted in a 1.4% reduction in HbA$_{1c}$ and a 59 mg/dl (3.3 mmol/l) reduction in fasting blood glucose levels when compared with placebo (19).

At a dose of 4 mg bid, rosiglitazone was associated with a reduction in fasting plasma glucose of 62 mg/dl (3.4 mmol/l) and reduction in HbA$_{1c}$ levels of 1.5% when compared with placebo (20).

Pioglitazone (30 mg/day) in combination with insulin resulted in a reduction in HbA$_{1c}$ of 1% and a reduction in fasting plasma glucose of 49 mg/dl (2.7 mmol/l). Unfortunately, studies on maximum doses of pioglitazone in combination with insulin have yet to be reported (19).

Combination Oral Therapy

Sulfonylurea/acarbose combination therapy has been reported to cause a 32 mg/dl (1.8 mmol/l) reduction in fasting plasma glucose when compared with sulfonylurea monotherapy. Additionally, postprandial glucose levels were 73 mg/dl (4 mmol/l) lower than those obtained with sulfonylurea monotherapy. Lastly, HbA_{1c} levels were 0.9% lower than in the sulfonylurea monotherapy group (21).

Sulfonylurea/metformin combination therapy has been reported to cause a 77 mg/dl (4.3 mmol/l) reduction in fasting plasma glucose and a 1.9% reduction in HbA_{1c} levels compared with sulfonylurea monotherapy (22).

Sulfonylurea/troglitazone therapy was reported to cause a 79 mg/dl (4.4 mmol/l) reduction in fasting plasma glucose and a 2.7% reduction in HbA_{1c} levels compared with sulfonylurea monotherapy. In this trial, troglitazone was administered at a dose of 600 mg/day (18). The addition of 300 mg/day of troglitazone to sulfonylurea therapy resulted in a mean reduction of HbA_{1c} and fasting blood glucose levels of 1.3% and 58 mg/dl (3.2 mmol/l), respectively. Although combination therapy with troglitazone is no longer an option, these studies show the effectiveness of combining sulfonylureas with glitazones.

When added to metformin therapy, repaglinide resulted in a further reduction in fasting plasma glucose levels and HbA_{1c} levels of 40 mg/dl (2.2 mmol/l) and 1.4%, respectively, compared with baseline treatment with metformin (6). Acarbose added to metformin therapy resulted in a reduction in fasting plasma glucose, postprandial glucose, and HbA_{1c} levels of 23 mg/dl (1.3 mmol/l), 62 mg/dl (3.4 mmol/l), and 0.8%, respectively, compared with metformin monotherapy (23). The addition of pioglitazone (30 mg/day) to metformin therapy resulted in a mean reduction of 0.8% in HbA_{1c} and 38 mg/dl (2.1 mmol/l) in fasting blood glucose levels when compared with placebo (19). A trial evaluating the addition of 8 mg/day of rosiglitazone to metformin therapy reported reductions in fasting plasma glucose and HbA_{1c} levels of 53 mg/dl (2.9 mmol/l) and 1.2%, respectively, when compared with placebo (20).

EFFECTS ON LIPIDS

Any medication that reduces blood glucose levels will probably be related to some indirect lowering of plasma lipid levels. However, some antihyperglycemic agents do have direct effects on plasma lipids. The sulfonylureas and repaglinide have no direct effect on levels of triglyceride, HDL cholesterol, or LDL cholesterol. Metformin has been associated with a slight reduction in triglyceride levels, a slight increase in

HDL cholesterol, and slight reductions in LDL cholesterol (–16%, 2%, and –8%, respectively) (1,11).

Acarbose has been associated with a slight reduction in triglycerides, LDL, and total cholesterol and a slight improvement in HDL cholesterol (1). Its greatest effect on lipid levels has been on triglycerides. In one study, triglyceride levels were reduced by 43 mg/dl (2.4 mmol/l) when compared with a 28 mg/dl (1.6 mmol/l) reduction observed with placebo (23). Pioglitazone monotherapy at a dose of 45 mg/day was associated with a 9.3% reduction in triglycerides, a 19.1% increase in HDL, and no consistent differences in LDL or total cholesterol when compared with treatment with placebo (19). In patients treated with 8 mg of rosiglitazone per day, free fatty acid levels were reduced by 14.7%, LDL cholesterol was increased by 18.6%, and HDL cholesterol was increased by 14.2% (20).

CONTRAINDICATIONS AND SIDE EFFECTS

Sulfonylureas and Meglitinides

The primary side effects of sulfonylureas are hypoglycemia and weight gain (1). In the UK Prospective Diabetes Study (UKPDS), patients in the intensive therapy arm treated with chlorpropamide gained 5.7 lb more than patients on conventional therapy. Patients treated with glyburide gained 3.8 lb more than those treated with conventional therapy (24).

Although in the past it was hypothesized that increases in insulin concentration in patients treated with sulfonylureas could lead to weight gain and possibly cardiovascular disease, it should be noted that the UKPDS concluded that sulfonylureas imparted no significant risk for the development of cardiovascular disease.

The incidence of hypoglycemia in patients treated with sulfonylureas is variable and depends on the specific agent used and the population evaluated. One trial revealed a 20% chance of hypoglycemia every 6 months in patients treated with sulfonylureas (2). In this particular review, severe hypoglycemia was reported most frequently with chlorpropamide and glyburide, followed by glipizide and finally first-generation sulfonylureas. Glimepiride is the latest sulfonylurea to be approved by the FDA and is the most potent. Because it has a duration of 24 h, it can be taken once daily. It has the lowest incidence of hypoglycemia and does not effect potassium channels in the heart.

Less common side effects of sulfonylureas include dermatological reactions, gastrointestinal disturbances, and hematological reactions (1). Antabuse-like (disulfiram) reactions and hyponatremia had been reported in patients using chlorpropamide (1). Acetohexamide and chlorpropamide should not be used in patients with renal dysfunction (1). Additionally, tolazamide and glyburide have partially active metabolites that may accumulate in patients with creatinine clearances of <30 ml/min. Glimepiride, glipizide, and tolbutamide are preferred for patients with moderate to severe renal dysfunction (1).

All of the sulfonylureas undergo hepatic metabolism and should therefore be used cautiously in patients with hepatic dysfunction (1).

The side effects of the meglitinides are virtually identical to those found with the sulfonylureas. Repaglinide is metabolized by oxidative transformation and conjugation with glucaronic acid to three major metabolites that have no pharmacological activity. Less than 2% of the parent drug is excreted unchanged in the feces, and less than 0.1% is excreted renally. Therefore, the compound is primarily metabolized in the liver and is excreted in the feces. Because of this metabolic pattern, repaglinide should be used cautiously and with longer intervals between doses in patients with hepatic dysfunction (1).

Efficacy trials have been scheduled in patients with renal dysfunction. Currently it is recommended that repaglinide be used cautiously and with longer intervals between doses in patients with renal dysfunction or in those on hemodialysis.

α-Glucosidase Inhibitors

The most common side effects of the α-glucosidase inhibitors are dose-related gastrointestinal complaints, abdominal pain, flatulence, and diarrhea. In many cases these side effects may be mitigated with continued administration of the drug and with slow stepwise titration.

Elevated hepatic enzymes have been reported at higher doses of acarbose (200 and 300 mg tid); however, the occurrence of hepatic dysfunction with doses of ≤100 mg tid is rare. In fact, elevated serum transaminase levels are no more frequent than those observed with placebo when doses of ≤100 mg tid were used (25).

One problem that may be encountered in patients treated with acarbose and hypoglycemic agents (e.g., insulin or sulfonylureas) is difficulty in treating hypoglycemic episodes with oral complex carbohydrates. The absorption rates of complex carbohydrates are drastically reduced with the administration of acarbose, so their use will not resolve hypoglycemia. Therefore, patients treated with α-glucosidase inhibitors and oral hypoglycemic agents should be advised to have a source of glucose such as glucose tablets or gel on hand in the event of a hypoglycemic episode (1).

Contraindications for the use of α-glucosidase inhibitors primarily revolve around gastrointestinal side effects. Acarbose should be avoided in patients with inflammatory bowel disease, colonic ulceration, or obstructive bowel disorders. Relative contraindications include medical conditions that might deteriorate with increased intestinal gas formation and chronic intestinal disorders of digestion or absorption (25).

Acarbose should be avoided in patients with serum creatinine levels >2.0 mg/dl.

Metformin

Patients treated with metformin may experience a 30% higher incidence of abdominal bloating, nausea, cramping, feeling of fullness, and diarrhea. These side effects can be a particular problem during the initiation phases of therapy. However, these side effects are usually self-limiting and transient and can be mitigated by starting with a low dose, titrating up slowly, and taking the medication with food (1).

Less common side effects include a reduction in cyanocobalamin levels (vitamin B_{12}) and a metallic taste in the mouth (1). Lactic acidosis can occur with the administration of metformin, but it is extremely rare (0.03 cases per 1,000 patient-years) and has occurred primarily in patients with significant renal dysfunction (17). Metformin is contraindicated in patients with renal dysfunction (serum creatinine >1.5 mg/dl in men, >1.4 mg/dl in women). This is due to the fact that metformin is excreted entirely unchanged via the kidneys and can accumulate in patients with significant renal dysfunction.

Metformin should be avoided in patients with congestive heart failure, unstable heart disease, hypoxic lung disease, or advanced age (>80 years). Because lactic acidosis is sometimes associated with hepatic dysfunction, metformin is contraindicated in patients with clinical or laboratory evidence of hepatic dysfunction. Metformin is also contraindicated in patients with a history of alcoholism or binge drinking and in patients with acute or chronic acidosis. Metformin should also be withheld temporarily in patients with acute conditions predisposing them to acute renal failure or acidosis, such as exacerbation of congestive heart failure, major surgical procedure, cardiovascular collapse, or acute myocardial infarction. Lastly, metformin should be discontinued just before the administration of intravenous iodinated contrast media and reinstituted 48 h or so after the procedure, after the patient's renal function has been verified (17).

Thiazolidinediones

Rosiglitazone and pioglitazone have been associated with mild to moderate edema in some patients. On the other hand, troglitazone was not associated with significantly more edema than placebo (18–20).

Thiazolidinediones are, however, contraindicated in patients with NYHA (New York Heart Association) class III and IV failure, since their safety in this population has not been established.

In phase III trials with troglitazone, slightly more than 2% of patients treated with medication had reversible elevations in AST and ALT greater than three times the upper limit of normal. On the other hand, no hepatic toxicity has yet been observed with either rosiglitazone or pioglitazone. Troglitazone was associated with several cases of fulminant hepatic failure resulting in death or the need for liver transplantation. Because of this, all thiazolidinediones require monitoring of liver function and are contraindicated in patients with liver function abnormalities.

Pioglitazone monotherapy has been associated with a 1.1- to 6.6-lb average weight increase compared with a 2.8- to 4.1-lb weight loss in patients treated with placebo (19). Rosiglitazone monotherapy has been associated with a 2.6- to 7.7-lb weight gain (20).

Reductions in hemoglobin and hematocrit have been observed in patients treated with pioglitazone and rosiglitazone. These changes are probably secondary to volume expansion and have not been associated with significant hematological effects. Because of this, no routine monitoring for anemia is recommended.

Insulin

The most significant side effects of insulin in patients with type 2 diabetes include hypoglycemia and weight gain. Severe hypoglycemia, while a major concern in patients with type 2 diabetes, probably occurs much less frequently than in patients with type 1 diabetes (26). In the metformin arm of the UKPDS at 10-year follow-up, 0.3% of patients treated with insulin/metformin had experienced a major hypoglycemic episode, and 34% of patients treated with just insulin had experienced milder hypoglycemic episodes (27).

Insulin has also been associated with significant weight gain. Studies in patients treated with insulin for between 6 and 12 months have reported weight gains of up to 6 kg (1).

Epidemiological studies have demonstrated a correlation between endogenous hyperinsulinemia and the risk of macrovascular disease. This has raised the question of whether insulin therapy accelerates macrovascular disease (26). However, it should be noted that the UKPDS concluded that insulin therapy was not associated with any increase or acceleration of macrovascular disease (24).

Note that with all medications used to treat diabetes, titration of doses is required to gain the maximum effect of the medication and to prevent or reduce side effects.

PATIENT ADHERENCE AND COST OF THERAPY

One of the most important considerations in the choice of a pharmacological regimen should be the expected degree of patient adherence to that regimen (28). One must always be concerned about the possibility of patient noncompliance because of side effects of the medication or because of difficulty in following the regimen. Adherence is a particular concern in patients with type 2 diabetes because they often must be treated with other medications to manage coexisting illnesses, such as hypertension, hyperlipidemias, cardiovascular abnormalities, and neuropathies. The addition of an antihyperglycemic agent or agents to an already complex regimen must be done in the most acceptable manner possible.

Recently, a ranking of the degree of patient adherence in patients managed with various antihyperglycemic agents was published in *Clinical Diabetes* (29). In this assessment, two major factors were considered: ease of use and discomforting side effects. According to this report, "ease of use of oral tablets and capsules is mainly governed by the number of daily doses needed" (29). It is widely accepted and well understood that compliance drops dramatically as the daily number of doses escalates. Additionally, discomforting side effects may limit patients' adherence to medication regimens. For example, it was reported in the UKPDS 3-year follow-up that a significant number of patients treated with chlorpropamide refused medications after they had experienced an ethanol-induced antibuse-like reaction (30).

Table 2.1 ranks the sulfonylureas, metformin, acarbose, and glitazones in relative terms of *1*) ease of use and *2*) discomforting side effects.

Table 2.1 Ease of Use and Patient Adherence to Hypoglycemic Medications

Medication	East of Use (0 = best, 4 = worst)	Common Discomforting Side Effects (0 = least, 5 = most)	Patient Adherence (0 = best, 9 = worst)
Sulfonylureas	1.5	1	2.5
Acarbose	3	3	6
Metformin	2.5	2	4.5
Glitazones	1	0	1

From White (29).

Table 2.2 Cost per Month (30-Day Supply) to the Pharmacist for Commonly Used Oral Antidiabetic Agents

Drug (Trade Name)	Usual Daily Dose (mg)	Cost in US$
First-generation sulfonylureas		
Acetohexamide	500–750	14.18
Chlorpropamide	250–375	14.69
Tolazamide	250–500	3.50
Tolbutamide	1–2,000	17.35
Second-generation sulfonylureas		
Glimepiride	1–4	7.34
Glipizide	10–20	21.93
Glucotrol XL	5	10.34
Glyburide	5–20	15.17–24.30
Micronized glyburide	3–12	17.61–21.31
Alpha-glucosidase inhibitors		
Acarbose	50–100	46.54
Miglitol	50–100	51.75
Thiazolidinediones		
Rosiglitazone	4–8	75.00–108.75
Pioglitazone	15–45	85.50
Others		
Metformin	1,500–2,550	54.35
Repaglinide	1–4	67.12

These two entities are then evaluated together to generate a numerical patient-adherence value. This value is a ranking from 0 to 9, with 0 being the best patient adherence and 9 being the worst patient adherence. Based on this ranking, the thiazolidinediones are the medications with the best adherence, followed by the sulfonylureas, metformin, and last, acarbose.

The cost of medication may also be considered in the choice of a regimen for a particular patient; however, cost should not be the primary driver in the clinician's choice of medication. It is difficult to assess cost comprehensively because of the great disparities in the cost of a medication to the patient from one region of the country to the other and the differences in cost to the patient between various insurance plans and health maintenance organizations. Table 2.2, which was adapted from the August 13, 1999 *Medical Letter* shows the cost per month to the pharmacist for commonly used oral agents. It is also widely known that the effect of a medication on the outcomes of diabetes care are not necessarily shown in the cost of treatment per day or per month.

TYPE 2 DIABETES TREATMENT ALGORITHMS

In 1995 it was relatively easy to develop a treatment algorithm for a type 2 diabetes patient. The patient could be placed on a program of diet and exercise and one of several sulfonylureas could be prescribed. As the type 2 diabetes progressed, the sulfonylureas would become less effective and insulin was then added, usually as an injection at bedtime. Then the FDA approved metformin, followed by acarbose and then troglitazone and eventually repaglinide and additional thiazolidinediones.

At present, the development of a meaningful, clinically effective, and relevant medication treatment regimen for type 2 diabetes is complex and providers do not find it easy to decide which medication to prescribe. The prescriber must consider the patient's weight, diabetes duration, lipid and blood pressure status, dexterity, and liver and kidney function, as well as the medications that have been tried previously. Fasting plasma glucose, HbA_{1c} levels, postprandial glucose levels, allergies, insurance coverage, cost of therapy, dosing complexity and the time it takes to titrate to effective doses, degree of insulin resistance, and whether or not the β-cell is still capable of producing and releasing insulin are all additional considerations. For these reasons, an exact step-by-step treatment algorithm is difficult to develop and various clinics follow different guidelines.

The type 2 diabetes treatment algorithm in Fig. 2.1 will allow you consider medication choices for patients with particular needs in addition to encouraging your patients to include a balanced nutrition and exercise program in their daily treatment regimen.

CONCLUSION

The hyperglycemia encountered in patients with type 2 diabetes is often accompanied by other metabolic abnormalities, such as hyperlipidemia, hyperinsulinemia, hypertension, and weight gain. In the past several years many new oral medications have been introduced that address not only glycemic abnormalities but also other metabolic abnormalities in patients with type 2 diabetes. While the cost of medication should be considered, the most effective method of achieving cost savings in the management of type 2 diabetes is via strict glycemic control with medications that do not adversely affect the patient's metabolic profile and do not carry contraindications to the patient's specific situation. When designing a therapeutic regimen for a given patient, the practitioner should consider the amount of glycemic lowering needed to bring that patient into glycemic control (achieving American Diabetes Association goals for treatment), the contraindications of the medication, the side

Patient has type 2 diabetes
according to American Diabetes Association criteria

CONSIDER the following:

Duration of diabetes
Degree of insulin resistance
Degree of obesity
Postprandial blood glucose
Is FPG >140 mg/dl?
Is HbA₁c >8% ?
Determine comorbidities
and other patient-care needs

At BASELINE, determine or implement the following:

HbA₁c
Serum creatinine, microalbuminuria
Blood pressure, body mass index, waist-to-hip ratio
Liver function tests
Lipid profile: HDL, LDL, total cholesterol, triglycerides
Cardiovascular risk
Have eyes examined for retinopathy
Determine if any neuropathies
Foot examination and training in preventative foot care
Have patient trained to self-monitor blood glucose daily
Refer for in-depth diabetes education
Prescribe daily aspirin therapy
Recommend daily micronutrient supplements

Start meal plan & aerobic exercise (20 min 3 days/week, unless
contraindicated because of complications) for ALL patients
(The only treatment for patients with initial FPG <200 mg/dl)

Figure 2.1 Drug Therapy Algorithm for Type 2 Diabetes

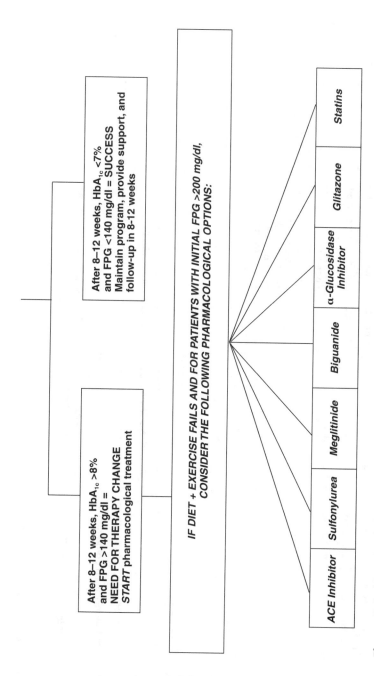

Figure 2.1 (*Continued*)

If patient is hypertensive, get BP to 135/80.	If patient is lean, start at lowest dose and titrate to effective maximum dose.	If patient is lean, has postprandial blood glucose elevations, use 30 min before each meal.	If patient is overweight, is dyslipidemic has high FPG, metformin is the drug of choice.	If patient is older and has postprandial blood glucose elevations, start with low dose and titrate over 10 weeks to maximum dose of 100 mg tid with the first bite of each meal.	If patient is insulin resistant, use either pioglitazone or rosiglitazone; titrate dose to maximum dose; evaluate liver function.	Use to normalize blood lipids.

*IF MONOTHERAPY DOES NOT ACHIEVE TREATMENT OBJECTIVES IN
3 MONTHS THEN ADD A SECOND ORAL AGENT.........*

Commonly used combinations include:

Sulfonylurea + Metformin   Sulfonylurea + Acarbose or Miglitol   Repaglinide + Metformin
Sulfonylurea + Glitazone   Glitazone + Metformin

Figure 2.1 (*Continued*)

IF INITIAL FPG LEVELS ARE >250–300 mg/dl, ASSUME GLUCOTOXICITY AND TREAT PATIENT WITH INSULIN LISPRO OR NPH INSULIN IN COMBINATION WITH AN ORAL AGENT.........

Commonly used combinations of insulin with oral agents include:

Sulfonylurea in the morning + NPH insulin at bedtime

Lispro insulin before meals + Sulfonylurea in the morning   Acarbose or Miglitol + NPH Insulin

Metformin + NPH insulin   Glitazone + NPH insulin

IF INITIAL FPG LEVELS ARE >400 mg/dl OR IF COMBINATION THERAPY FAILS, SWITCH TO INSULIN THERAPY (0.3–0.5 U/kg ideal body wt).........

Commonly used insulin regimens include:

NPH twice daily with two-thirds in the morning and one-third before dinner

NPH mixed with regular or lispro insulin twice daily

Lispro or regular insulin before meals and NPH or ultralente at bedtime

Use of lispro insulin in an insulin pump

Figure 2.1 (*Continued*)

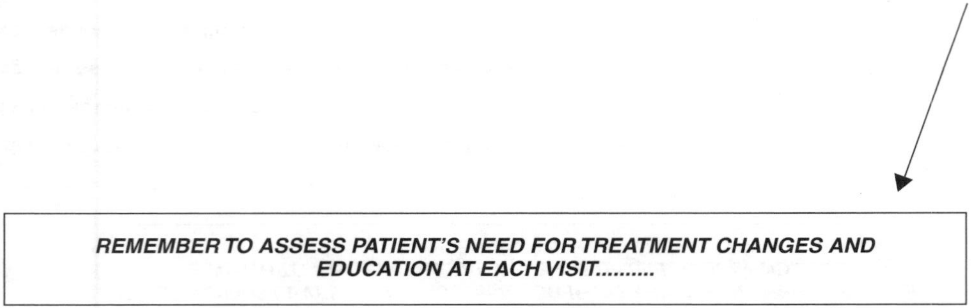

REMEMBER TO ASSESS PATIENT'S NEED FOR TREATMENT CHANGES AND EDUCATION AT EACH VISIT........

Adapted from Campbell RK: Type 2 diabetes mellitus: disease state management. *Primary Care Special Edition* 3:35, 1999. FPG, fasting plasma glucose; BP, blood pressure.

Figure 2.1 (*Continued*)

effects of the medication, the effect of the medication on insulin resistance, the expected degree of patient adherence, and lastly, medication costs. Clinicians presently have an expanded medication tool chest from which to select drug therapy that will allow achievement of metabolic objectives and still allow patients a flexible and near-normal lifestyle.

REFERENCES

1. White JR: The pharmacological reduction of blood glucose in patients with type 2 diabetes mellitus. *Clin Diabetes* 16:58–67, 1998

2. Gerich JE: Oral hypoglycemic agents. *N Engl J Med* 321:1232–1245, 1989

3. Kolterman OG: Longitudinal evaluation of the effects of sulfonylurea therapy in subjects with type 2 diabetes mellitus. *Am J Med* 79:23–33, 1985

4. Vinambres C, Villanueva-Penacarilo ML, Valverde I, Malaisse WJ: Repaglinide preserves nutrient-stimulated biosynthetic activity in rat pancreatic islets. *Pharmacol Res* 34:83–85, 1996

5. Gromada J, Dissing S, Kofod H, Frokjaer-Jensen J: Effects of hypoglycemic drugs repaglinide and glibenclamide on ATP-sensitive potassium channels and cytosolic calcium levels in beta TC3 cells and rat pancreatic beta cells. *Diabetologia* 38:1025–1032, 1995

6. Prandin (repaglinide) package insert, NovoNordisk, 1999

7. Damsbo P, Anderson PH, Lund S, Porksen N: Improved glycemic control with repaglinide in NIDDM with 3 times daily meal related dosing (Abstract). *Diabetes* 46 (Suppl. 1):34A, 1997

8. Dagogo-Jack S, Santiago JV: Pathophysiology of type 2 diabetes and modes of action of therapeutic interventions. *Arch Intern Med* 157:1802–1817, 1997

9. White J: The pharmacologic management of patients with type II diabetes mellitus in the era of new oral agents and insulin analogs. *Diabetes Spectrum* 9:227–234, 1996

10. Yu JG, Kruszynska YT, Mulford MI, Olefsky JM: A comparison of troglitazone and metformin on insulin requirements in euglycemic intensively insulin-treated type 2 diabetic patients. *Diabetes* 48:2414–2421, 1999

11. DeFronzo RA: Pharmacologic therapy for type 2 diabetes mellitus. *Ann Intern Med* 131:281–303, 1999

12. Santeusanio F, Compagnucci P: A risk-benefit appraisal of acarbose in the management of non-insulin-dependent diabetes mellitus. *Drug Safety* 11:432–444, 1994

13. Saltiel AR, Olefsky JM: Thiazolidinediones in the treatment of insulin resistance and type II diabetes. *Diabetes* 45:1661–1669, 1996

14. Pugh JA, Wagner ML, Sawyer J, Ramirez G, Tuley M, Friedberg SJ: Is combination sulfonylurea and insulin therapy useful in NIDDM patients? A meta-analysis. *Diabetes Care* 15:953–959, 1992

15. Johnson JL, Wolf SL, Kabadi UM: Efficacy of insulin and sulfonylurea combination therapy in type II diabetes: a meta-analysis of randomized, placebo-controlled studies. *Arch Intern Med* 156:259–264, 1996

16. Genuth S: Insulin use in NIDDM. *Diabetes Care* 13:1240–1264, 1990

17. Glucophage (metformin) package insert, Bristol-Meyers Squibb, 1999

18. Rezulin (troglitazone) package insert, Parke-Davis, 1999

19. Actos (pioglitazone) package insert, Ely Lilly, 1999

20. Avandia (rosiglitazone) package insert, SmithKline Beecham, PA, 1999

21. Chiasson J-L, Josse RG, Hunt JA, Palmason C, Rodger NW, Ross SA, Ryen EA, Tan MH, Wolevert MS: The efficacy of acarbose in the treatment of patients with non-insulin-dependent diabetes mellitus. *Ann Intern Med* 121:928–935, 1994

22. Gugliano D, Quatraro A, Consoli G, Minei A, Ceriello A, DeRosa N, Onofrio ED: Metformin for obese, insulin-treated diabetic patients: improvement in glycaemic control and reduction of metabolic risk factors. *Eur J Clin Pharmacol* 44:107–112, 1993

23. Coniff RF, Shapior JA, Seaton TB, Bray G: Multicenter, placebo-controlled trial comparing acarbose (BAYg5421) with placebo, tolbutamide, and tolbutamide-plus-acarbose in non-insulin-dependent diabetes mellitus. *Am J Med* 98:443–451, 1995

24. UK Prospective Diabetes Study (UKPDS) Group: Intensive blood glucose control with sulfonylureas or insulin compared with conventional treatment and risk of complications in patients with type 2 diabetes (UKPDS 33). *Lancet* 352:837–852, 1998

25. Precose (acarbose) package insert, Bayer Pharmaceuticals, 1999

26. Genuth S: Insulin use in NIDDM. *Diabetes Care* 13:1240–1264, 1990

27. UK Prospective Diabetes Study (UKPDS) Group: Effect of intensive blood glucose control with metformin on complications in overweight patients with type 2 diabetes (UKPDS 34). *Lancet* 352:854–865, 1998

28. White JR: The cost of managing diabetes mellitus: focus on the oral pharmacologic management of type II diabetes. *J Managed Care Pharm* 5:113–120, 1999

29. White J: Combination of oral agents/insulin therapy in patients with type II diabetes mellitus. *Clin Diabetes* 15:102–113, 1997

30. UK Prospective Diabetes Study Group: United Kingdom Prospective Diabetes Study (UKPDS) 13: relative efficacy of randomly allocated diet, sulphonylurea, insulin, or metformin in patients with newly diagnosed noninsulin dependent diabetes followed for three years. *BMJ* 310:83–88, 1995

3. Sulfonylureas

Quick Reference

Sulfonylureas: Six sulfonylurea agents are currently available in the U.S.:
chlorpropamide (Diabinese [Pfizer] and generic formulations),
tolbutamide (generic), tolazamide (generic), glyburide (glibenclamide; Diabeta [Hoechst Marion Roussel]), glipizide (Glucotrol
[Pfizer]), and glimepiride (Amaryl [Hoechst Marion Roussel]).
Mechanism of Action: The sulfonylureas exert their blood glucose–
lowering effect in patients with type 2 diabetes by stimulating
insulin secretion at the level of the pancreatic β-cell. They are also
thought to exert extrapancreatic effects that appear to improve the
metabolic pathways involved in type 2 diabetes.
Pharmacokinetics: All sulfonylureas are completely absorbed; however,
these drugs differ substantially in their onset and duration of action.
All sulfonylureas are also metabolized in the liver. The first-
generation agents are excreted exclusively by renal mechanisms,
whereas the newer agents are excreted in both urine and bile.
Dosage Forms and Dose:

Table 3.1

Drug	Dosage Forms
Chlorpropamide	100- and 250-mg tablets
Tolbutamide	500-mg tablets
Tolazamide	250- and 500-mg tablets
Glyburide (Glibenclamide)	2.5- and 5-mg tablets
Glipizide and Glipizide GITS	5- and 10-mg tablets and 2.5-, 5- and 10-mg tablets
Glimepiride	1-, 2-, and 4-mg tablets

Table 3.2

Sulfonylurea	Usual Starting Dose	No. of Daily Doses	Dose Titration	Usual Maintenance Dose
Chlorpropamide	250 mg daily	1	50–125 mg at intervals of 3–5 days	100–500 mg daily; usually 250 mg daily
Tolbutamide	1–2 g daily as divided doses	3	Adjusted according to patient response	0.25–3 g daily; maximum of 3 g
Tolazamide	100–250 mg daily with breakfast or first main meal	1–2	100–250 mg at intervals of 1 week	250–500 mg daily with breakfast; if >500 mg needed, divide into two daily doses
Glyburide (Glibenclamide)	1.5–5 mg daily with breakfast or first main meal	1–2	2.5 mg at intervals of 1 week	1.25–20 mg daily as a single dose or in divided doses; maximum of 20 mg daily
Glipizide	5 mg before breakfast	1–2	2.5–5 mg at intervals of at least several days	15 mg once daily; doses >15 mg as divided doses; maximum total daily dose of 40 mg
Glipizide GITS	2.5–10 with breakfast	1	2.5 mg at intervals of at least a week	2.5–20 mg daily
Glimepiride	1–2 mg daily with breakfast or first main meal	1	No more than 2 mg at intervals of 1–2 weeks	1–4 mg daily; maximum of 8 mg daily

Special Populations: All sulfonylureas should be used with caution in patients with hepatic dysfunction. Chlorpropamide is contraindicated in patients with renal impairment. These agents should be used with caution in the elderly and other individuals at increased risk of hypoglycemia.

Precautions and Adverse Effects: Sulfonylureas are ineffective in patients with diabetic ketoacidosis, type 1 diabetes, or known hypersensitivity to sulfonylureas. The most common adverse effect is hypoglycemia. Hypoglycemia may occur more frequently in patients with hepatic, adrenal, or pituitary insufficiency, as well as in elderly, debilitated, or malnourished patients. Other adverse effects, including gastrointestinal disturbances, are uncommon.

INTRODUCTION

Sulfonylureas have been used in the management of type 2 diabetes for more than 40 years (1,2). Their mechanism of action in reducing hyperglycemia is complex, but essentially, they act on the pancreatic β-cell to increase both basal and meal-stimulated insulin secretion. Some studies have suggested sulfonylureas exert minor effects through extrapancreatic mechanisms. Long-term glycemic control with sulfonylurea treatment can cause improvement in several metabolic pathways in type 2 diabetes, including decreased overproduction of hepatic glucose, improved insulin action in skeletal muscle and adipose tissue, and increased efficiency of meal-stimulated insulin secretion.

Six sulfonylurea agents are currently available in the U.S.: the first-generation agents chlorpropamide, tolbutamide, and tolazamide; and the second-generation agents glyburide (glibenclamide), glipizide, and glimepiride.

PHARMACOLOGY

Mechanism of Action

Sulfonylureas exert their antihyperglycemic effect by stimulating insulin secretion in the pancreas (1). Insulin secretion is regulated by ATP-dependent potassium channels in the plasma membrane of the pancreatic β-cell (2). The ATP-dependent potassium channel consists of two subunits, one containing a sulfonylurea receptor and the other containing the channel itself. In patients with type 2 diabetes who retain some degree of β-cell function, sulfonylureas bind to the sulfonylurea receptor and close the ATP-dependent potassium channel. As potassium accumulates within the β-cell membrane, the β-cell depolarizes, leading to an influx of calcium. The increased concentration of calcium causes insulin granules to migrate to the cell surface, where the granules rupture and release the insulin.

Sulfonylureas are also thought to exert extrapancreatic effects on the liver, peripheral tissues, and skeletal muscle (1). Although the precise mechanisms by which these effects improve hyperglycemia have not been demonstrated, it is likely that the direct effect of insulin secretion by the pancreas results in portal hyperinsulinemia that suppresses hepatic glucose production and causes a decrease in fasting plasma glucose. The improved glycemic state ameliorates glucose toxicity, thereby enhancing insulin sensitivity in skeletal muscle and adipose tissue. Patients with type 2 diabetes characteristically have defects in both insulin secretion and insulin action; therefore, regardless of the mechanism of action of the sulfonylurea drugs, they are effective in controlling hyperglycemia in these patients.

Pharmacokinetics

The sulfonylureas display marked differences in absorption, metabolism, and elimination (1). The first-generation sulfonylureas (chlorpropamide, tolbutamide, and tolazamide) are extensively protein bound, whereas the second-generation agents (glyburide or glibenclamide, glipizide, and glimepiride) do not bind to circulating plasma proteins.

All sulfonylureas are nearly completely absorbed; however, the onset and the duration of action are determined by the unique pharmacokinetic features of each agent and its specific formulation (1,2). Most sulfonylureas have a relatively short plasma half-life, usually in the range of 4–10 h; only chlorpropamide has a half-life longer than 24 h (Table 3.3). Because most sulfonylureas maintain glycemic control effectively with twice-daily dosing, the tissue half-life on the β-cell receptor must be considerably longer than the plasma half-life.

All sulfonylureas are metabolized in the liver, some to weakly active or inactive metabolites, others, such as chlorpropamide, only partially (1,2). The first-generation sulfonylureas are excreted exclusively by the kidney, whereas the second-generation agents and their metabolites are excreted in differing proportions in the urine and feces (1). A higher proportion of biliary excretion occurs with glyburide and glimepiride than with glipizide (2).

INDICATIONS

Sulfonylureas are indicated as an adjunct to nutrition therapy and exercise to lower blood glucose levels in patients with type 2 diabetes whose hyperglycemia has not been controlled adequately by nutrition therapy

Table 3.3 Comparative Pharmacokinetics of Sulfonylureas

Sulfonylurea	Dose Range (mg)	Peak Level (h)	Duration of Effect (h)	Half-Life (h)	Metabolites	Excretion
Tolbutamide	500–3,000	3–4	6–10	5–7	Inactive	Urine
Chlorpropamide	100–500	2–4	36–48	24–48	Active or unchanged	Urine
Tolazamide	100–1,000	3–4	16–24	7	Weakly active	Urine
Glipizide	2.5–40	1–3	12–14	2–4	Inactive	Urine 80% Feces 20%
Glyburide	1.25–20	~4	12–24	10	Inactive and weakly active	Urine 50% Feces 50%
Glimepiride	1–8	2–3	16–24	9	Active	Urine 60% Feces 40%

From Groop and DeFronzo (1) and Lebovitz (2).

alone (2,3). The ideal candidates for treatment with sulfonylureas are patients with type 2 diabetes who have significant insulin deficiency but sufficient residual β-cell function to respond to stimulation (2). Patients are likely to demonstrate a good glycemic response to sulfonylureas if they (1,2)

- had onset of hyperglycemia after age 30 years
- have been diagnosed with hyperglycemia for <5 years
- have a fasting glucose level <300 mg/dl (16.7 mmol/l)
- are normal weight or obese
- are willing to comply with a reasonable nutrition and exercise program
- are not totally insulin deficient

Sulfonylureas should be administered to patients with type 2 diabetes whose blood glucose has not been adequately controlled by a 4- to 6-week trial of appropriate nutrition therapy (2). Nutrition therapy must be continued after the addition of the sulfonylurea. Patients presenting with marked symptoms and random plasma glucose levels of ~300 mg/dl (16.7 mmol/l) may best be started on nutrition and sulfonylurea therapy simultaneously (2). However, many patients with newly diagnosed diabetes who have random plasma glucose levels >300 mg/dl (16.7 mmol/l) are best initially treated with insulin and instruction in appropriate nutrition, because the deleterious effects of glucose toxicity and their level of insulin deficiency makes them unlikely to achieve acceptable glycemic control (1,2). After a 1- to 6-week intensive course of insulin therapy plus nutrition therapy to achieve adequate glycemic control (fasting plasma glucose <120–140 mg/dl (6.7–7.8 mmol/l), sulfonylurea treatment may be able to replace insulin therapy.

Treatment with sulfonylureas is typically instituted at a low dose and increased at 4- to 7-day intervals until the maximal benefit is achieved (1,2). The goal of sulfonylurea therapy is to maintain fasting and preprandial blood glucose levels between 80 and 120 mg/dl (4.4 and 6.7 mmol/l) and an HbA_{1c} of <7%. In patients with good dietary compliance and in those who lose weight, sulfonylurea therapy may be reduced or discontinued; however, some data suggest that maintenance therapy with low doses of a sulfonylurea can better provide long-term glycemic control.

Most patients will achieve the maximal benefit in improved glycemic control with one-half to two-thirds of the recommended maximal dose (1,2). When sulfonylurea therapy fails to meet target blood glucose levels (<140 mg/dl [7.8 mmol/l]), a second oral antihyperglycemic agent can be added to the regimen.

Approximately 20–25% of patients with newly diagnosed type 2 diabetes fail to respond to initial sulfonylurea therapy (primary failures) and are best treated with another oral antihyperglycemic agent (1,3). Of the 75–80% of patients who initially achieved good glycemic control, 3–5% lose their responsiveness each year (secondary failures), most likely because of progressive β-cell failure, tachyphylaxis to the sulfonylurea, and dietary noncompliance.

INSTITUTING SULFONYLUREA THERAPY

A number of factors influence the choice of a sulfonylurea, including its intrinsic potency, onset of action, duration of action, patterns of metabolism and excretion, and beneficial and detrimental side effects (2). The intrinsic potency of a sulfonylurea is a function of its binding affinity to the receptor (2). Glyburide and glimepiride are the most potent drugs in this class, and tolbutamide is the least potent. Glimepiride does not affect potassium channels in cardiac tissue and has been shown to have extrapancreatic effects that reduce the incidence of hypoglycemia.

Dosage Forms

One of the characteristics of type 2 diabetes is the delayed and diminished secretion of meal-stimulated insulin, which results in an early and excessive increase in postprandial blood glucose levels (2). Therefore, the more rapid the onset of action of a sulfonylurea, the shorter the delay in the rise of postprandial glucose. The timing of the sulfonylurea dose should be such that the peak of insulin secretion coincides with the peak postprandial glucose level. (See Table 3.1).

Dosage and Administration (4–9)

The duration of action of a sulfonylurea is an important consideration (2,3). (See Table 3.2.) Of the first-generation agents, chlorpropamide has a very long half-life and duration of action and needs to be given only once daily; tolbutamide, on the other hand, has a very short duration of action and needs to be administered two or three times a day. Most of the second-generation agents, which have a duration of 16–24 h, can be administered once a day at the usual therapeutic doses, but maximal doses may need to be divided into two daily doses. A newer second-generation agent, glimepiride, may be administered before or with breakfast, with equivalent blood glucose–lowering effect (10).

The degree and frequency of severe hypoglycemic reactions associated with sulfonylurea treatment appear to be related to duration of action (3). Therefore, a shorter-acting sulfonylurea may be preferable for certain patients, such as the elderly, those with poor nutrition, patients who are likely to miss meals, or those with hepatic, renal, or cardiovascular disease, to minimize the risk of hypoglycemia (see Special Populations below).

The patterns of metabolism and excretion are also important to the risk of side effects (2,3). Because sulfonylureas are metabolized, and therefore inactivated, in the liver, the risk of hypoglycemia is significantly increased in patients with hepatic impairment. Similarly, sulfonylureas that are excreted primarily in the urine are more likely to cause hypoglycemia in patients with renal dysfunction than are those that are excreted in large part via the biliary tract.

THERAPY WITH SULFONYLUREAS IN COMBINATION WITH OTHER ANTIHYPERGLYCEMIC AGENTS

When a particular sulfonylurea fails to maintain acceptable glycemic control, the treatment options include the use of a sulfonylurea in combination with another oral agent or with insulin (3). Not all combination regimens of sulfonylureas with other oral agents or insulin are approved by the U.S. Food and Drug Administration.

The rationale for combination therapy lies in the mechanism of action of sulfonylureas, to increase insulin secretion. As insulin secretory function declines because of progressive β-cell failure, a sulfonylurea has a diminished effect on insulin secretion. The mechanisms by which other oral antihyperglycemic agents reduce blood glucose levels can complement the action of sulfonylureas to achieve glycemic control.

For example, the combination of a sulfonylurea and metformin is effective because metformin does not affect β-cell function; rather, it reduces hepatic glucose production and improves insulin resistance in skeletal muscle, providing an additive glucose-lowering effect (11). Sulfonylurea/metformin combinations are the most commonly used oral combination therapy for type 2 diabetes.

α-glucosidase inhibitors delay the absorption of glucose in the small intestine. When added to a sulfonylurea, these agents provide an additive effect by lowering postprandial glucose levels and improving the action of endogenous insulin (11).

The thiazolidinediones also enhance insulin sensitivity in skeletal muscle and glucose utilization in the liver, and several clinical trials have demonstrated their effectiveness as combination therapy with a sulfonylurea (11).

Sulfonylureas and insulin have been used extensively in combination therapy (3). Glycemic control can usually be achieved with this combination by the addition of insulin in a relatively low dose administered in a simple regimen. The extrahepatic effects of the sulfonylurea are thought to increase the efficacy of the insulin. One of the more successful regimens involves the administration of bedtime insulin in combination with daytime sulfonylurea, often referred to as BIDS therapy (1,3).

SPECIAL POPULATIONS

Patients with Hepatic or Renal Dysfunction

Because sulfonylureas are metabolized in the liver, they are, as a class, contraindicated in patients with hepatic dysfunction (1). Chlorpropamide is contraindicated in patients with diminished renal function because the kidney is the primary mode of excretion (1).

Elderly Patients

Hypoglycemia is the most significant risk of the use of sulfonylureas and other oral agents in elderly patients (12). Both renal and hepatic insufficiency are substantial risk factors for the development of severe hypoglycemia during sulfonylurea treatment in the elderly. Chlorpropamide is contraindicated in elderly patients (>60–65 years) because of the normal age-related decline in glomerular filtration rate (1).

CONTRAINDICATIONS

The sulfonylureas are contraindicated in patients with a known hypersensitivity to the drug and in those with diabetic ketoacidosis (DKA), with or without coma. DKA should be treated with insulin (4–9).

WARNINGS

The product information for the sulfonylurea drugs contains a special warning that the administration of oral antidiabetic agents has been reported to be associated with increased risk of cardiovascular mortality compared with treatment with nutrition therapy alone or nutrition therapy plus insulin (4–9). This warning is based on the results of a long-term, prospective clinical trial, the University Group Diabetes Program (UGDP) (13). Although only one sulfonylurea, tolbutamide, was included in this study, this warning may also apply to other agents of this class, considering their similar modes of action and chemical structures. The validity of this finding has been questioned, however; the recent UK Prospective Diabetes Study (UKPDS) found no increased cardiovascular mortality with sulfonylureas (14).

PRECAUTIONS

Fasting blood glucose levels should be monitored periodically to determine the therapeutic response to sulfonylureas (4–9). HbA_{1c} concentrations should be monitored, usually every 3–6 months, to assess long-term glycemic control more precisely.

Hypoglycemia

The most serious complication of sulfonylurea therapy is hypoglycemia, and all sulfonylureas are capable of producing severe hypoglycemia (2–9). Appropriate patient selection, dosage, and instructions are important to avoid hypoglycemic episodes. Debilitated or malnourished patients and those with adrenal, pituitary, or hepatic insufficiency are particularly susceptible to the hypoglycemic action of sulfonylureas. Hypoglycemia may be difficult to recognize in the elderly and in people taking β-adrenergic blocking agents or other sympatholytic drugs. Hypoglycemia is more likely to occur when caloric intake is deficient, after severe or prolonged exercise, when alcohol is ingested, or when more than one glucose-lowering drug is used.

Loss of Blood Glucose Control

A loss of blood glucose control may occur if a patient experiences stress through fever, trauma, infection, or surgery (2–9). It may be necessary to institute insulin therapy in combination with the sulfonylurea. However, the combined use of a sulfonylurea and insulin may increase the risk of hypoglycemia.

Pregnancy and Nursing

The sulfonylureas are categorized in pregnancy category C (2–9). Chlorpropamide has not been evaluated for teratogenic effects. Glipizide and glimepiride have been found to be fetotoxic in rats at doses that produced maternal hypoglycemia. In some studies in rats, nonteratogenic skeletal deformities were observed after exposure during gestation and lactation. There are no adequate and well-controlled studies of sulfonylureas in pregnant women. On the basis of animal studies, sulfonylureas should not be used during pregnancy. Because a higher incidence of congenital abnormalities is associated with abnormal maternal blood glucose levels during pregnancy, insulin therapy is recommended during pregnancy to maintain blood glucose levels as close to normal as possible.

Pediatric Use

The safety and effectiveness of sulfonylureas in pediatric patients has not been established.

ADVERSE EFFECTS AND MONITORING

Sulfonylureas are usually well tolerated and the frequency of side effects, other than hypoglycemia, is low (1). The most common adverse events associated with sulfonylurea treatment are dizziness, headache, asthenia, and nausea (4–9). In comparative clinical trials, common adverse events occurred at similar incidences with glimepiride and glipizide but were less likely to occur with glimepiride than glibenclamide (10). Hematological complications, including thrombocytopenia, agranulocytosis, and hemolytic anemia have been described with tolbutamide and chlorpropamide but appear to be very rare with the second-generation sulfonylureas (1). Skin reactions are nonspecific and rare. Abnormal liver function tests and icterus are uncommon.

Certain side effects are unique to the specific agents because of their individual chemical structures (2,3). For example, chlorpropamide has antidiuretic properties that can lead to water retention and hyponatremia. In predisposed individuals, chlorpropamide frequently causes an alcohol-induced flush; this phenomenon also occurs occasionally with tolbutamide.

DRUG INTERACTIONS

The hypoglycemic action of sulfonylureas may be potentiated by certain drugs, including nonsteroidal anti-inflammatory agents and other drugs that are highly bound to protein, such as salicylates, sulfonamides, chloramphenicol, coumarins, probenecid, monoamine oxidase inhibitors, and β-adrenergic blocking agents (2–9). Patients given these drugs concomitantly with a sulfonylurea should be monitored closely for hypoglycemia. Similarly, when these drugs are withdrawn, patients on sulfonylurea therapy should be observed closely for loss of glycemic control.

Other drugs tend to produce hyperglycemia and may lead to loss of glycemic control in patients taking sulfonylureas. These drugs include the thiazides and other diuretics, corticosteroids, phenothiazines, thyroid products, estrogens, oral contraceptives, phenytoin, nicotinic acid, sympathomimetics, and isoniazid. When these drugs are withdrawn, patients should be observed closely for hypoglycemia.

CLINICAL EFFECT

As initial treatment in patients with type 2 diabetes, sulfonylureas can induce a mean decrease in HbA_{1c} of 1–2% and can reduce fasting plasma glucose by 60–70 mg/dl (3.3–3.8 mmol/l) (2). The improvement in glycemic control that occurs with sulfonylureas, as with other anti-diabetic agents, is somewhat greater in patients with less glycemic control and somewhat less in patients with only moderate hyperglycemia.

Approximately one-third of patients will achieve target glycemic goals with a regimen of a sulfonylurea plus nutrition therapy and exercise (2). Glycemic control will improve substantially in another third, but achievement of glycemic targets will require the addition of other antihyperglycemic agents. The remaining third of patients will not respond to sulfonylurea treatment and will require another therapeutic approach.

With the progressive decline in β-cell function, the response to sulfonylurea treatment diminishes over time, and changes in treatment strategy will be necessary (2). The decrease in β-cell function is not the only possible cause of a lack of effectiveness, however. An increase in insulin resistance may play a role. There are also patient-related factors, including weight gain, poor compliance, inactivity, and stress or intercurrent illness. Therapy-related factors are another possible reason for a lack of response; for example, inadequate dosage, impaired absorption due to hyperglycemia, and concomitant treatment with diabetogenic drugs.

REFERENCES

1. Groop LC, DeFronzo RA: Sulfonylureas. In *Current Therapy of Diabetes Mellitus.* DeFronzo RA, Ed. St. Louis, MO, Mosby, 1998, pp. 96–101

2. Lebovitz HE: Insulin secretagogues: sulfonylureas and repaglinide. In *Therapy for Diabetes Mellitus and Related Disorders.* 3rd ed. Lebovitz HE, Ed. Alexandria, VA, American Diabetes Association, 1998, pp. 160–170

3. Lebovitz HE: Oral antidiabetic agents. In *Joslin's Diabetes Mellitus.* Kahn CR, Weir GC, Eds. Philadelphia, Lea & Febiger, 1994, pp. 508–529

4. Diabinese (chlorpropamide) package insert, Pfizer, 1999

5. Orinase (tolbutamide) package insert, The Upjohn Company, 1993

6. Tolazamide at PlanetRx. PlanetRx.com. Health at Your Fingertips. Available at http://www.planetrx.com. Accessed September 39, 1999

7. Diabeta (glyburide) package insert, Hoechst Marion Roussel, 1996

8. Glucotrol (glipizide) package insert, Pfizer, 1999

9. Amaryl (glimepiride) package insert, Hoechst Marion Roussel, 1999

10. Langtry HD, Balfour JA: Glimepiride: a review of its use in the management of type 2 diabetes mellitus. *Drugs* 55:563–584, 1998

11. DeFronzo RA: Pharmacologic therapy for type 2 diabetes mellitus. *Ann Intern Med* 131:281–303, 1999

12. Halter JB: Geriatric patients. In *Therapy for Diabetes Mellitus and Related Disorders*. 3rd ed. Lebovitz HE, Ed. Alexandria, VA, American Diabetes Association, 1998, pp. 234–240

13. Meinert CL, Knatterud GL, Prout TE, Klimt CR: A study of the effects of hypoglycemic agents on vascular complications in patients with adult-onset diabetes. II. Mortality results. *Diabetes* 19 (Suppl. 2):789–830, 1970

14. UK Prospective Diabetes Study Group: Intensive blood glucose control with sulphonylureas or insulin compared with conventional treatment and risk of complications in patients with type 2 diabetes (UKPDS 33). *Lancet* 352:837–853, 1998

4. α-Glucosidase Inhibitors

Quick Reference

α-Glucosidase Inhibitors: Acarbose (Precose, Bayer Pharmaceuticals) and
miglitol (Glyset, Pharmacia & Upjohn/Bayer Pharmaceuticals) are
the two α-glucosidase inhibitors currently available in the U.S. for
treatment of type 2 diabetes.

Mechanism of Action: α-glucosidase inhibitors delay the absorption of
complex carbohydrates in the lower intestines, resulting in a blunting of the sharp rise in postprandial glucose levels associated with
digestion of a meal.

Pharmacokinetics: Following oral administration, very little of acarbose
is absorbed by the small intestines (bioavailability of 1–2%),
whereas miglitol is almost completely absorbed. Because both
drugs exert their effects locally, effect is not related to systemic
absorption. Absorbed drug is completely excreted in the urine,
while unabsorbed drug is excreted in the feces.

Dosage Forms and Dose:

Table 4.1

Drug Name	Dosage Forms
Acarbose	25-, 50-, and 100-mg tablets
Miglitol	25-, 50-, and 100-mg tablets

Table 4.2

Drug Name	Initial Dose*	Maximum Dose	Usual Maintenance Dose
Acarbose	25 mg tid	For patients ≤60 kg: 50 mg tid; for patients >60 kg: 100 mg tid	50 mg tid
Miglitol	25 mg tid	100 mg tid	50 mg tid

*Some patients may need to begin with once-daily dosing to decrease the likelihood of adverse effects.

Special Populations: Patients with renal dysfunction should not receive α-glucosidase inhibitors because drug accumulation could result. α-glucosidase inhibitors can be used at the normal dose in patients with hepatic dysfunction. They can also be administered at normal doses in elderly patients and without regard to sex or ethnicity. There is no information on the treatment of children with α-glucosidase inhibitors.

Precautions and Side Effects: The α-glucosidase inhibitors do not cause hypoglycemia, but may increase the risk of hypoglycemia when taken with oral sulfonylureas or insulin. Patients being treated with α-glucosidase inhibitors need to treat a hypoglycemic event with glucose tablets because absorption of dietary sugar, which can consist of complex carbohydrates, will be delayed. Gastrointestinal side effects, such as flatulence, abdominal pain, and bloating, are the most common side effects of α-glucosidase inhibitors. These side effects tend to be transient in nature and can be reduced with a lower initial dose and a slow titration schedule.

INTRODUCTION

The gold standard for measuring consistent euglycemia over a period of time is the glycated hemoglobin (HbA_{1c}) level. The primary components that affect HbA_{1c} are fasting plasma glucose (FPG) and postprandial plasma glucose (PPG) levels. In patients in whom control of PPG levels is difficult, HbA_{1c} levels will continue to be higher despite well-controlled FPG levels. More recent evidence suggests that poorly controlled PPG levels are a risk factor for coronary heart disease. Whether this risk is increased by high PPG levels, the resultant increase in postprandial insulin (PPI) levels, or a combination of both is not known, but the need to control high PPG levels in patient with diabetes is evident (1).

In the last few years, several new classes of antidiabetic medications have become available that are designed to decrease PPG and subsequent PPI levels. Among these are the α-glucosidase inhibitors, which act by delaying the absorption of simple carbohydrates in the small intestine, thereby blunting the PPG peak normally associated with the ingestion of a meal. Two of these medications, acarbose (Precose, Bayer Pharmaceuticals) and miglitol (Glyset, Pharmacia & Upjohn/Bayer Pharmaceuticals), are approved for use in the U.S.

PHARMACOLOGY

Mechanism of Action

α-glucosidase inhibitors are named for their ability to reversibly bind α-glucosidase enzymes in the brush border of the small intestine. These enzymes include sucrase, maltase, isomaltase, and glucoamylase. α-glucosidase enzymes assist in the digestion of dietary carbohydrates by breaking down disaccharides and oligosaccharides (i.e., sugar and starch) into glucose and other monosaccharides that can be absorbed in the small intestine. The competitive, reversible binding by the α-glucosidase inhibitors delays the absorption of carbohydrates from the gastrointestinal tract, which results in more even absorption of simple sugars throughout the gut. This results in the blunting of the normally sharp rise in PPG levels associated with the digestion of a meal (2–4).

The affinity that acarbose and miglitol have for α-glucosidase enzymes differs somewhat. Miglitol does not have an inhibitory effect on lactase, whereas acarbose inhibits a small percentage (~10%); however, this percentage is small enough that lactose absorption is not affected (3). Acarbose also inhibits pancreatic amylase, whereas miglitol does not (4–6). In addition, miglitol appears to be a more potent inhibitor than acarbose on a milligram-to-milligram basis (2,5,6). There is no evidence that these differences in affinity or potency have any significant clinical effects.

There has been some speculation in the clinical literature of a second mechanism of action for miglitol. Unlike acarbose, miglitol is almost completely absorbed by the small intestine, leading researchers to consider an additional, extraintestinal effect of the drug. Specifically, miglitol has been shown to have a suppressive activity on hepatic glycogenolysis in vitro (7), which is theorized to occur in vivo as well. Several studies have been conducted to explore the possibility of an extraintestinal effect of miglitol that could lower FPG levels secondary to suppressing glycogenolysis (8–11). The results are contradictory, so it is not possible to draw any conclusions about the clinical significance of this alternative mechanism of action. It should be noted, however, that the manufacturer of miglitol states that "there is no evidence that systemic absorption of miglitol contributes to its therapeutic effect" (4).

Pharmacokinetics

Acarbose. Following oral administration of acarbose, very little of the drug is absorbed by the small intestine. The bioavailability of the active drug is ~1–2%, and peak plasma concentrations occur in ~1 h. In addition, metabolites formed from intestinal bacteria and gut enzymes breaking down the drug have a bioavailability of ~34%, with absorption occurring ~14–24 h after drug administration.

As described above, metabolism of acarbose occurs exclusively in the intestines. The natural bacterial flora and digestive enzymes break acarbose down into at least 13 different metabolites. Only one metabolite appears to have α-glucosidase–inhibiting behavior. The small amount of unchanged drug that is absorbed is completely excreted renally (12–14).

Miglitol. Following oral administration of miglitol, peak plasma concentrations normally occur in ~3 h. Miglitol is absorbed from the small intestine via an active transport mechanism that represents a rate-limiting step and can affect both the bioavailability of the drug and the timing of its onset of action. Both vary in accordance with the amount of the drug administered. At a dose of 25 mg, the absorption is rapid and complete, with a bioavailability of ~100%. At higher doses, such as the maximum recommended dose of 100 mg, complete absorption can take up to 7 h, with bioavailability values ranging from 50 to 70%. Because the site of action of miglitol is the brush border of the small intestine, the absorption rate of the drug does not affect its clinical efficacy.

Miglitol is primarily distributed into extracellular fluids, with minimal tissue penetration. This results in the relatively small volume of distribution of 0.18 l/kg. Miglitol has very low permeation of the blood-brain barrier. Protein binding of miglitol is <4%. Miglitol is renally excreted unchanged, with any drug not initially absorbed in the small intestine being eliminated in the feces. No metabolism of miglitol is observed. The amount excreted in the urine is directly affected by the amount absorbed via the active transport mechanism in the small intestines. As such, the amount of renal excretion is correlated with the initial dosage administered. At lower doses, such as 25 mg, the amount excreted unchanged in the urine is 95%. At higher doses, such as

100 mg, the amount excreted unchanged in the urine is less, representing ~95% of the incompletely absorbed drug. The elimination half-life is 2–3 h (4,15).

INDICATIONS

Acarbose has been approved by the U.S. Food and Drug Administration (FDA) as monotherapy for type 2 diabetes in patients whose diabetes is not well-controlled with nutrition therapy alone. Acarbose has also been approved for combination therapy with sulfonylureas, insulin, or metformin (14). Miglitol has been approved by the FDA as monotherapy for type 2 diabetes in patients whose diabetes is not well-controlled with nutrition therapy alone or in combination with oral sulfonylureas (4).

DOSING CONSIDERATIONS

Dosage Forms

For a list of dosage forms, see Table 4.1 (4,14).

Dosage and Administration

Treatment for diabetes must be individualized for each patient to assure maximal clinical efficacy with minimal adverse effects. (See Table 4.2.) The incidence of gastrointestinal side effects can be significantly reduced for patients receiving α-glucosidase inhibitors by starting with a small initial daily dose and titrating slowly to an appropriate maintenance dose. All doses should be given with the first bite of each meal, since α-glucosidase inhibitors can only exert their effects in the presence of dietary carbohydrates in the small intestines (4,14).

Many patients may experience reduced gastrointestinal side effects by using an acarbose dosing regimen that starts with an initial dose of 25 mg qd for 2 weeks, followed by 25 mg bid for 2 weeks, and then 25 mg tid. Once a patient is tolerating 25 mg tid, the titration schedule for acarbose is to increase the dose by 50 mg tid every 4–8 weeks, depending on 1-h PPG levels, HbA_{1c}, and adverse effects. The titration schedule for miglitol is 25 mg tid for 4–8 weeks, followed by 50 mg tid for 3 months, at which time efficacy should be assessed with an HbA_{1c} measurement. Patients who are not adequately responding to miglitol therapy and who are tolerant of a higher dose can then be increased to 100 mg tid (4,14).

SPECIAL POPULATIONS

Renal Dysfunction

Systemically absorbed α-glucosidase inhibitors are almost exclusively eliminated renally. Therefore, drug accumulation can occur in patients with renal dysfunction, particularly with miglitol, given its high amount of systemic absorption compared with acarbose (4,14).

Hepatic Dysfunction

There is no need for dose adjustments of α-glucosidase inhibitors for patients with hepatic dysfunction. α-glucosidase inhibitors are not hepatically metabolized, and their pharmacokinetics are not altered in patients with cirrhosis (4,16).

Elderly

There is no need for dose adjustments of α-glucosidase inhibitors for elderly patients. No significant differences in pharmacokinetics have been observed in elderly patients versus younger patients for either drug (4,14). The clinical effect of miglitol in treating elderly patients has been studied (see Clinical Effect below).

Pediatrics

No information regarding the treatment of children with α-glucosidase inhibitors is available.

Ethnicity

No information on the pharmacokinetics of acarbose in different ethnic groups is available. One U.S. clinical study showed similar clinical efficacy in European-American and African-American patients, with a slightly better trend in Hispanic-American patients (4). The pharmacokinetics of acarbose are similar in Caucasian and Japanese patients, and its pharmacodynamics are similar in Caucasian and African-American patients (14). The clinical effect of miglitol in treating African-American and Hispanic patients has been studied (see Clinical Effect below).

Sex

No information is available on treating men versus women with acarbose. There are no significance differences in the pharmacokinetics of miglitol between men and women (4).

CONTRAINDICATIONS

Acarbose and miglitol are both contraindicated in patients with the following conditions (4,14):

- Diabetic ketoacidosis
- Gastrointestinal problems
    □ Inflammatory bowel disease
    □ Colonic ulceration
    □ Partial intestinal obstruction
    □ Chronic intestinal diseases associated with marked disorders of digestion or absorption or with conditions that may deteriorate as a result of increased gas formation in the intestine
- Hypersensitivity to acarbose or miglitol or any of their components

In addition, acarbose is contraindicated in patients with cirrhosis or with a plasma creatinine concentration of >2.0 mg/dl (176.8 (mol/L) (14). Although miglitol is not specifically contraindicated in patients with renal dysfunction, its use is not recommended because renal dysfunction can result in a high systemic accumulation of the drug (4).

PRECAUTIONS

Hypoglycemia

α-glucosidase inhibitors do not cause hypoglycemia, but when used in combination with oral sulfonylureas or insulin, hypoglycemia may result. Because α-glucosidase inhibitors block the absorption of dietary carbohydrates, patients experiencing hypoglycemia must use glucose tablets instead of foods containing complex carbohydrates to raise blood glucose levels. In the case of severe hypoglycemia, a glucagon injection or intravenous glucose injections may be necessary (4,14).

Loss of Control of Blood Glucose

Patients must remember to monitor blood glucose levels, particularly in stressful situations such as fever, infection, trauma, or surgery, all of which can raise blood glucose levels regardless of treatment with α-glucosidase inhibitors. Treatment with insulin may be necessary in these situations to avoid diabetic ketoacidosis (4,14).

Renal Impairment

Since α-glucosidase inhibitors are primarily excreted renally, these agents should not be used in patients with renal impairment or insufficiency (i.e., creatinine clearance <25 ml/min) (4,14).

Pregnancy and Nursing

Acarbose and miglitol are both pregnancy category B, indicating that the safety of the drug has not been established in pregnant women. Both drugs are excreted in small amounts in breast milk, so neither is recommended as treatment in nursing mothers (4,14)

Pediatrics

No information is available regarding the treatment of children with α-glucosidase inhibitors (4,14).

SIDE EFFECTS AND MONITORING

Gastrointestinal

The adverse effects of α-glucosidase inhibitors occur secondary to their innate mechanism of action. Both acarbose and miglitol exert their action locally in the small intestine, blocking the breakdown and absorption of complex carbohydrates. The delayed absorption results in the complex sugars moving to the large intestine. The natural flora of the large intestine ferment the carbohydrates, resulting in the production of gas, which leads to the most common side effects of α-glucosidase inhibitors: flatulence, abdominal distention and pain, and diarrhea (4). The gastrointestinal effects are by far the most common problem associated with α-glucosidase inhibitors, occurring in one- to two-thirds of patients receiving acarbose in clinical trials (17–19). The incidence of similar problems in patients treated with miglitol tends to be a bit lower (20–27), but this could be due to the use of lower initial doses and appropriate dose titration in these trials.

The gastrointestinal symptoms of α-glucosidase inhibitors tend to be transient in nature. Redistribution of the digestive enzymes in the gut usually occurs several weeks after therapy is initiated, resolving the common adverse effects (18). The delayed carbohydrate absorption caused by α-glucosidase inhibitors does not result in significant weight loss or malnutrition problems in patients taking the drug on a long-term basis (28–30).

Hepatic

Elevated liver function tests (i.e., transaminases) have been observed in clinical trials with patients taking acarbose at dosages of 200–300 mg tid. All enzyme elevations resolved with the discontinuation of therapy (31,32). Elevated liver function tests have only been observed in patients receiving dosages of acarbose that exceed the manufacturer's recommended maximum dose of 100 mg tid (18,19). The manufacturer of acarbose recommends monitoring liver functions tests every 3 months during the first year of treatment and periodically thereafter. Dose reductions or discontinuation may be necessary if elevation of liver function tests occurs (14).

DRUG INTERACTIONS

As described in the Precautions section above, an additive hypoglycemic effect may occur when α-glucosidase inhibitors are used in combination with sulfonylureas or insulin. Several studies of combination therapy with α-glucosidase inhibitors and insulin have shown a decreased need for insulin, sometimes requiring a reduction in insulin dosage to avoid a hypoglycemic event (18,19,33–35). Any medications that elevate glucose levels, including thiazide diuretics, corticosteroids, oral contraceptives and estrogen, niacin, phenothiazides, thyroid supplements, and calcium-channel blockers, may reduce the efficacy of α-glucosidase inhibitors (4,14).

Miglitol has been shown to reduce the AUC (area under the curve) and peak concentrations of glyburide, but the clinical significance of this interaction is unknown. A similar interaction occurs with metformin, but the reduction is minimal (4). Acarbose has no effect on the absorption and distribution of glyburide (14). Acarbose does cause a significant reduction in the acute bioavailability of metformin, but overall bioavailability is not affected, so there is most likely no clinical significance to this interaction (36).

Acarbose has no interactions with digoxin, nifedipine, propanolol, or ranitidine (4). Acarbose has been shown to elevate liver function tests at very high doses, so it might be prudent to avoid acetaminophen, a well-known hepatic toxin, if a patient drinks alcohol regularly (37). Results from studying interactions between digoxin and miglitol have been contradictory, showing a reduction of digoxin levels in healthy volunteers but not in patients with diabetes (4). The reason for this discrepancy is unknown, but providers may wish to consider monitoring digoxin levels periodically in patients taking these two drugs concomitantly. Miglitol also significantly reduces the bioavailability of propanolol and ranitidine, but has no drug interactions with nifedipine, antacids, or warfarin (4,38). Activated charcoal and digestive enzyme preparations, such as amylase and pancreatin, may interfere with the local activity of α-glucosidase inhibitors in the gut (4,14).

CLINICAL EFFECT

There have been over 200 clinical trials performed measuring the clinical efficacy of acarbose. Acarbose was used extensively in Europe long before its FDA approval in the U.S. Miglitol boasts a somewhat more modest number of studies. The clinical efficacies of acarbose and miglitol appear to be similar; however, no comparative clinical trials have been conducted, so it is difficult to judge whether there is any clinical advantage to using one product versus the other.

Several large clinical trials with acarbose, including the large post-marketing PROTECT (Precose Resolution of Optimal Titration to Enhance Current Therapies) study, which enrolled over 6,000 patients, have shown a decrease in HbA_{1c} values of ~0.5–0.7%, or ~0.6–1.1% when baseline changes in placebo-treated patients are subtracted from baseline changes in acarbose-treated patients. PPG levels tend to decrease in the range of 40–50 mg/dl (2.2–2.8 mmol/l), and FPG decreases in the range of 25–30 mg/dl (1.4–1.7 mmol/l) (39,40).

Small short-term studies and larger clinical trials have shown the primary clinical effects of miglitol to be a modest decrease in HbA_{1c} levels, a significant decrease in PPG levels, and a subsequent small decrease in PPI levels. Mean placebo-subtracted changes in HbA_{1c} from baseline range from 0.4% to 1.2% in the larger trials, with the notable exception of one study that measured a change of 1.3%. PPG levels have a large range of change, decreasing by ~20–60 mg/dl (1.1–3.3 mmol/l). There is a unique collection of studies in the miglitol clinical literature that address specific patient populations with a high prevalence of diabetes: Hispanic-American, African-American, and elderly patients. Results of these studies are similar to those described above (20–27).

REFERENCES

1. Mooradian AD, Thurman JE: Drug therapy of postprandial hyper-glycaemia. *Drugs* 57:19–29, 1999

2. Taylor RH, Barker HM, Bowey EA, Canfield JE: Regulation of the absorption of dietary carbohydrate in man by two new glycosidase inhibitors. *Gut* 27:1471–1478, 1986

3. Bischoff H: Pharmacology of alpha-gluconidase inhibition. *Eur J Clin Invest* 24 (Suppl. 3):3–10, 1994

4. Glyset (miglitol) package insert, Pharmacia & Upjohn, 1998

5. Madar Z: The effect of acarbose and miglitol (BAY-m-1099) on post-prandial glucose levels following ingestion of various sources of starch by nondiabetic and streptozotocin-induced diabetic rats. *J Nutr* 119:2023–2029, 1989

6. Madar Z, Hazan A: Effect of miglitol and acarbose on starch diges-tion, daily plasma glucose profiles and cataract formation. *J Basic Clin Pharmacol* 4:69–81, 1993

7. Bollen M, Stalmans W: The antiglycogenolytic action of 1-deoxyno-jirimycin results from a specific inhibition of the α-1,6-gluconidase activity of the debraching enzyme. *Eur J Biochem* 181:775–780, 1989

8. Joubert PH, Foukaridis GN, Bopape ML: Miglitol may have a blood glucose lowering effect unrelated to inhibition of alpha-glucosidases. *Eur J Clin Pharmacol* 31:723–724, 1987

9. Joubert PH, Venter HL, Foukaridis GN: The effect of miglitol and acarbose after an oral glucose load: a novel hypoglycaemic mecha-nism? *Br J Clin Pharmacol* 30:391–396, 1990

10. Sels JPJE, Kingma PJ, Wolffenbuttel BHR, Menheere PPCA, Branolte JH, Nieuwenhuijzen Kruseman AC: Effect of miglitol (BAY m-1099) on fasting blood glucose in type 2 diabetes mellitus. *Netherlands J Med* 44:198–201, 1994

11. Sels JPJE, Nauta JJP, Menheere PPCA, Wolffenbuttel BHR, Nieuwenhuijzen Kruseman AC: Miglitol (Bay m 1099) has no extraintestinal effects on glucose control in healthy volunteers. *Br J Clin Pharmacol* 42:503–506, 1996

12. Ahr HJ, Boberg M, Krause HP, Maul W, Muller FO, Ploschke HJ, Weber H, Wunsche C: Pharmacokinetics of acarbose. I. Absorption, concentration in plasma, metabolism and excretion after single

administration of [14C]acarbose to rats, dogs and man. *Arzneimittelforschung* 39:1254–1260, 1989

13. Ahr HJ, Krause HP, Siefert HM, Steinke W, Weber H: Pharmacokinetics of acarbose. II. Distribution to and elimination from tissues and organs following single or repeated administration of [14C] acarbose to rats and dogs. *Arzneimittelforschung* 39:1261–1267, 1989

14. Precose (acarbose) package insert, Bayer Pharmaceuticals, 1995

15. Ahr HJ, Boberg M, Brendal E, Krause HP, Steinke W: Pharmacokinetics of miglitol: absorption, distribution, metabolism, and excretion following administration to rats, dogs and man. *Arzneim Forsch/Drug Res* 47:734–745, 1997

16. Zillikens MC, Swart GR, van den Berg JW, Wilson JH: Effects of the glucosidase inhibitor acarbose in patients with liver cirrhosis. *Aliment Pharmacol Ther* 3:453–459, 1989

17. Krentz AJ, Ferner RE, Bailey CJ: Comparative tolerability profiles of oral antidiabetic agents. *Drug Safety* 11:223–241, 1994

18. Hollander P: Safety profile of acarbose, an alpha-glucosidase inhibitor. *Drugs* 44 (Suppl. 2):47–53, 1992

19. Reuser AJJ, Wisselaar HA: An evaluation of the potential side-effects of alpha-glucosidase inhibitors used for the management of diabetes mellitus. *Eur J Clin Invest* 24 (Suppl. 3):19–24, 1994

20. Pagano G, Marena S, Corgiat-Mansin L, Cravero F, Giorda C, Bozza M, Rossi CM: Comparison of miglitol and glibenclamide in diet-treated type 2 diabetic patients. *Diabete Metab* 21:162–167, 1995

21. Mitrakou A, Tountas N, Raptis AE, Bauer RJ, Schulz H, Raptis SA: Long-term effectiveness of a new α-glucosidase inhibitor (BAY m1099-miglitol) in insulin-treated type 2 diabetes mellitus. *Diabetic Med* 15:657–660, 1998

22. Segal P, Feig PU, Schernthaner G, Ratzmann KP, Rybka J, Petzinna D, Berlin C: The efficacy and safety of miglitol therapy compared with glibenclamide in patient with NIDDM inadequately controlled by diet alone. *Diabetes Care* 20:687–691, 1997

23. Johnston PS, Coniff RF, Hoogwerf BJ, Santiago JV, Pi-Sunyer FX, Krol A: Effects of the carbohydrase inhibitor miglitol in sulfonylurea-treated NIDDM patients. *Diabetes* Care 17:20–29, 1994

24. Escobar-Jiménez F, Barajas C, De Leiva A, Cano FJ, Masoliver R, Herrera-Pombo JL, et al.: Efficacy and tolerability of miglitol in

the treatment of patients with non-insulin-dependent diabetes mellitus. *Curr Ther Res* 56:258–268, 1995

25. Johnston PS, Lebovitz HE, Coniff RF, Simonson DC, Raskin P, Munera CL: Advantages of α-glucosidase inhibition as monotherapy in elderly type 2 diabetic patients. *J Clin Endocrinol Metab* 83:1515–1522, 1998

26. Johnston PS, Feig PU, Coniff RF, Krol A, Kelley DE, Mooradian AD: Chronic treatment of African-American type 2 diabetic patients with α-glucosidase inhibition. *Diabetes Care* 21:416–422, 1998

27. Johnston PS, Feig PU, Coniff RF, Krol A, Davidson HA, Haffner SM: Long-term titrated-dose α-glucosidase inhibition in non-insulin-requiring Hispanic NIDDM patients. *Diabetes Care* 21:409–415, 1998

28. Toeller M: Nutritional recommendations for diabetic patients and treatment with alpha-glucosidase inhibitors. *Drugs* 44 (Suppl. 3):13–20, 1992

29. Van-Gall L, Nobels F, De Leeuw I: Effects of acarbose on carbohydrate metabolism, electrolytes, minerals and vitamins in fairly well-controlled non-insulin-dependent diabetes mellitus. *Gastroenterol* 29:642–644, 1991

30. Tuonilehto J, Pohjola M, Lindstrom J, Aro A: Acarbose and nutrient intake in non-insulin dependent diabetes mellitus. *Diabetes Res Clin Pract* 26:215–222, 1994

31. Coniff RF, Shapiro JA, Robbins D, Kleinfield R, Seaton TB, Beisswenger P, McGill JB: Reduction of glycosylated hemoglobin and postprandial hyperglycemia by acarbose in patients with NIDDM: a placebo-controlled dose-comparison study. *Diabetes Care* 18:817–824, 1995

32. Coniff RF, Shapiro JA, Seaton TB, Bray GA: Multicenter, placebo-controlled trial comparing acarbose (BAY g 5421) with placebo, tolbutamide, and tolbutamide-plus-acarbose in non-insulin-dependent diabetes mellitus. *Am J Med* 98:443–451, 1995

33. Scheen AJ, Lefebvre PJ: Antihyperglycaemic agents: drug interactions of clinical importance. *Drug Safety* 12:32–45, 1995

34. Dimitriadis G, Hatziagellaki E, Alexopoulos E, Kordonouri O, Komesidou V, Ganotakis M, Raptis S: Effects of α-glucosidase inhibition on meal glucose tolerance and timing of insulin administration in patients with type I diabetes mellitus. *Diabetes Care* 14:393–398, 1991

35. Kennedy FP, Gerich JE: A new alpha-glucosidase inhibitor (Bay-m-1099) reduces insulin requirements with meals in insulin-dependent diabetes mellitus. *Clin Pharmacol Ther* 42:455–458, 1987

36. Scheen AJ, Ferreira Alves de Magalhaes AC, Salvatore T, Lefebvre PJ: Reduction of the acute bioavailability of metformin by the alpha-glucosidase inhibitor acarbose in normal man. *Eur J Clin Invest* 24 (Suppl. 3):50–54, 1994

37. Krahenbuhl S: Acarbose and acetaminophen: a dangerous combination? *Hepatology* 29:285–287, 1999

38. Schall R, Muller FO, Hundt HKL, Duursema L, Groenewoud G, Middle MV: Study of the effect of miglitol on the pharmacokinetics and pharmacodynamics of warfarin in healthy males. *Arzneim Forsch/Drug Res* 46:41–46, 1996

39. Campbell LK, White JR, Campbell RK: Acarbose: its role in the treatment of diabetes mellitus. *Ann Pharmacother* 30:1255–1262, 1996

40. Buse J, Hart K, Minasi L: The PROTECT study: final results of a large multicenter postmarketing study in patients with type 2 diabetes: Precose Resolution of Optimal Titration to Enhance Current Therapies. *Clin Ther* 20:257–269, 1998

5. Glitazones

Quick Reference

Thiazolidinediones: Two thiazolidinediones are currently available in the U.S.: rosiglitazone (Avandia, SmithKline Beecham) and pioglitazone (Actos, Eli Lilly). These drugs are sometimes referred to as insulin sensitizers.

Mechanism of Action: These drugs reduce insulin resistance and improve blood glucose levels, probably via the stimulation of peroxisome-proliferator-activated receptor-gamma (PPARγ). They not only affect glycemic control but can also alter lipid levels.

Pharmacokinetics: Pioglitazone and rosiglitazone are well absorbed without regard to meals. These drugs are extensively metabolized.

Dosage Forms and Dose:

Table 5.1

Drug	Dosage Forms
Rosiglitazone	2-, 4-, and 8-mg tablets
Pioglitazone	15-, 30-, and 45-mg tablets

Table 5.2

	Initial Dose (mono-therapy)	Initial Dose (Cmb with insulin)	Initial Dose (Cmb with metformin)	Initial Dose (Cmb with sulfonylurea)	Maximum Dose	Titration Interval
Rosiglitazone	2 mg bid or 4 mg qd	N/A	2 mg bid or 4 mg qd	N/A	4 mg bid or 8 mg qd	12 weeks
Pioglitazone	15–30 mg qd	15–30 mg qd	15–30 mg qd	15–30 mg qd	45 mg qd	4 weeks*

Cmb, combination therapy.
* Interval not specifically recommended in the package insert but used in the cited phase III trials.

Special Populations: These drugs can be administered in usual doses to patients with renal dysfunction, to the elderly, to any ethnic group, and without regard to sex. However, these drugs should not be used in patients with hepatic dysfunction.

Precautions and Side Effects: These drugs can worsen hypoglycemia in patients taking insulin or sulfonylureas. Resumption of ovulation may occur in anovulatory premenopausal females taking thiazolidinediones. Minor reductions in hematocrit and hemoglobin may occur. Mild to moderate edema is reported in some patients treated with thiazolidinediones. The thiazolidinediones should usually be avoided in patients with New York Heart Association (NYHA) class III and IV heart failure. Mild weight gain and edema may occur in patients treated with thiazolidinediones. Patients being managed with thiazolidinediones should have their hepatic function monitored.

INTRODUCTION

The first thiazolidinedione, ciglitazone, was synthesized in 1982 (1). It was soon thereafter discovered that ciglitazone reduced insulin resistance in obese and diabetic animals. Because of their effects on insulin resistance, thiazolidinediones have been developed as pharmacological agents for the management of type 2 diabetes, although they were initially synthesized as potential lipid-reducing agents. Since their discovery, three thiazolidinediones have been introduced to the market in the U.S.: troglitazone (Rezulin) (2), rosiglitazone (Avandia) (3), and pioglitazone (Actos) (4). In March 2000, troglitazone was withdrawn from the market because of liver toxicity.

These compounds are orally active and are unrelated to the other oral agents either chemically or by mechanism of action. A thiazolidine-2,4-dione structure is common to all three of these drugs, with differences in potency, receptor binding, metabolic effects, pharmacokinetics, and side effects being governed by modifications in the side chain. They have been used in the management of type 2 diabetes as monotherapeutic agents and in combination with insulin, metformin, and suflonylureas. Additionally, they have been studied and found to be effective in treating insulin-resistant women with polycystic ovarian syndrome (5). These agents are sometimes referred to as "insulin sensitizers" (6).

PHARMACOLOGY

Mechanism of Action

The precise mechanism of action or relative importance of various mechanisms of action of the thiazolidinediones is not completely understood. These drugs improve glycemic control by increasing insulin sensitivity (3). The primary mechanism of action appears to be the direct stimulation of a family of receptors on the nuclear surface of cells that are responsible for the modulation of lipid homeostasis, adipocyte differentiation, and insulin action. Thiazolidinediones are potent and highly selective agonists for one of the isoforms in this family of receptors, known as peroxisome-proliferator-activated receptor-gamma (PPARγ) (2–4). The thiazolidinediones also display some cross reactivity with other isoforms in the PPAR family, PPARα and PPARδ (7–8). Different relative affinities of various thiazolidinediones for these three receptor types may explain the different effects these three agents have on lipid profiles.

PPARγ is probably the most important of these three receptors in terms of the antidiabetic action of thiazolidinediones. A relationship between ability to stimulate PPARγ and antihyperglycemic activity has been reported (7). Thiazolidinediones stimulate the expression of genes responsible for the production of glucose transporters (GLUT1 and GLUT4). PPARγ stimulation has also been shown to reduce TNF-α (tumor necrosis factor alpha) and hepatic glucokinase expression (7). Thiazolidinediones may cause a reduction in the number of large adipocytes and an increase in the number of small adipocytes, leading to lower free fatty acid and triglyceride levels and improved insulin sensitivity. The relative importance of each of these mechanisms or potential mechanisms is not currently understood.

Pharmacokinetics

Pioglitazone (4). After the administration of pioglitazone, maximum concentration (C_{max}) occurs within 2 h. Food may delay the absorption rate but not the extent of absorption. Pioglitazone may be taken without regard to meals. Pioglitazone is extensively bound to serum protein (>99%), whereas its metabolites M-III and M-IV are >98% bound. The apparent volume of distribution (Vd) is a mean of 0.63 L/kg. Pioglitazone is extensively metabolized via oxidation and hydroxylation, with metabolites being partially converted to glucoronide or sulfate conjugates. Metabolites M-III (keto derivatives) and M-IV (hydroxy derivatives), along with parent pioglitazone, are the predominant species found in human serum at steady state. Approximately 15–30% of pioglitazone can be recovered in the urine following oral administration. The mean serum half-lives of pioglitazone and total pioglitazone are 3–7 h and 16–24 h, respectively. Pioglitazone clearance is 5–7 L/h.

Rosiglitazone (3). Following the administration of rosiglitazone, C_{max} occurs within 1 h. Food may delay the absorption rate, but the extent of absorption is not clinically significantly changed. Rosiglitazone may be taken without regard to meals. It is extensively bound to serum protein (>99.8%), primarily albumin. The apparent volume of distribution (Vd) was a mean of 17.6 L/kg in the population studied. Rosiglitazone is extensively metabolized via *N*-demethylation and hydroxylation, followed by conjugation with glucoronic acid or sulfate. No unchanged drug is found in the urine. The metabolites of rosiglitazone are less potent than the parent compound and are not thought to contribute to the insulin-sensitizing effects of the drug. After administration of labeled rosiglitazone, ~64% is eliminated via the urine and 23% is eliminated via the feces. The mean serum half-life for labeled rosiglitzone material ranges from 103 to 158 h. Rosiglitazone clearance is ~3 L/h.

INDICATIONS

Currently, rosiglitazone is approved for monotherapeutic use and in combination with metformin (3). Troglitazone is approved for combination use with insulin, metformin, or sulfonylureas or for triple combination therapy (2). Pioglitazone is approved for monotherapeutic use and for combination therapy with metformin, sulfonylureas, or insulin (4).

DOSING CONSIDERATIONS

Dosage Forms

See Table 5.1 for information on dosage forms.

Dosage and Administration

See Table 5.2 for dosage and administration information. Please note that pioglitazone can always be given just once daily, usually in the morning. Rosiglitazone is given either once or twice daily.

SPECIAL POPULATIONS

Renal Dysfunction

Dose adjustments for rosiglitazone or pioglitazone are not required in patients with renal dysfunction (2–4). However, use of some of the other antihyperglycemic agents is not recommended in patients with renal dysfunction, thereby eliminating the possibility of combination therapy with those agents (combination metformin/thiazolidinedione therapy, for example) in this population.

Hepatic Dysfunction

Patients with impaired hepatic function (Child-Pugh grade B/C) have a 45% reduction in pioglitazone and total pioglitazone mean peak concentrations, but no change in mean area under the curve (AUC) when compared with normal subjects. In patients with impaired hepatic function (Child-Pugh grade B/C), C_{max} and AUC values for rosiglitazone were increased two- and threefold, respectively, and elimination half-life was increased by 2 h. Rosiglitazone and pioglitazone should not be used in patients with clinical evidence of active liver disease or with serum ALT concentrations >2.5 times the upper limit of normal (3,4).

Elderly

Age does not result in clinically significant changes in the effects or pharmacokinetics of rosiglitazone or pioglitazone. No dosage adjustment are needed in this population (2–4).

Pediatric

No pharmacokinetic, safety, or efficacy data for the thiazolidinediones is available in children. Seldom, if ever, would this class of medications be physiologically reasonable to use in a pediatric population.

Ethnicity

No differences in the effects of these agents has been observed in any ethnic group.

Sex

Plasma concentrations of troglitazone and its metabolites are similar among male and female patients (2). However, the mean C_{max} and

AUC values for pioglitazone have been found to be 20–60% higher in female subjects than in male subjects. Mean reductions were generally greater (0.5%) in female subjects than in male subjects (4). Rosiglitazone clearance was reported to be 6% lower in males of comparable body weight (3). In monotherapeutic trials with rosiglitazone, a slightly greater therapeutic response (quantitative differences were not reported) was observed in female patients, while no such difference was reported in metformin/rosiglitazone combination trials. Interestingly, sex-related differences were less marked in more obese patients. Women tend to have a greater fat mass than men for a given body mass index (BMI). The sex-related differences in effect may be due to this difference in fat mass because the molecular target PPARγ is highly expressed in lipid tissue (3). Although there are slight differences in the effects of both rosiglitazone and pioglitazone in women, no dose adjustment is recommended and, as in men, treatment in women must be individualized.

CONTRAINDICATIONS

The thiazolidinediones are contraindicated in patients with known hypersensitivity to thiazolidinediones or any component of the products and in patients with liver disease (2–4).

PRECAUTIONS

Diabetes

These agents should not be used to treat patients with type 1 diabetes or to manage patients in diabetic ketoacidosis (2–4).

Hypoglycemia

Patients whose diabetes is being managed with a thiazolidinedione in combination with insulin or oral hypoglycemic agents may be at risk for hypoglycemia. In some cases, a reduction in the dose of the hypoglycemic agent may be warranted (2–4).

Ovulation

The thiazolidinediones may cause resumption of ovulation in premenopausal women with anovulation secondary to insulin resistance. These patients may be at risk for pregnancy if adequate contraception is not used (2–4). Thiazolidinediones have been studied as a treatment for anovulation in women with polycystic ovarian syndrome and have been shown to be effective (5).

Hematology

Reductions in hemoglobin and hematocrit have been observed in patients treated with pioglitazone and rosiglitazone. Reductions in hemoglobin and hematocrit with the thiazolidinediones are ≤4% and ≤1 g/dl, respectively (2–4). These changes are possibly due to volume expansion and have not been associated with significant hematological effects. They occur within the first 4–8 weeks of therapy and have been shown to persist for at least 2 years (2–4).

Edema

Rosiglitazone and pioglitazone have been associated with mild to moderate edema in some patients (3,4).

Cardiac

In the phase III trials of rosiglitazone and pioglitazone, patients with New York Heart Association (NYHA) class III and IV status were excluded because troglitazone had adverse cardiac effects in animal studies and because it was known that thiazolidinediones can cause volume expansion and therefore increased preload. Patients with class I and II failure were studied via serial echocardiography, and no changes in cardiac size or function were observed. Thiazolidinediones are contraindicated in patients with NYHA class III and IV failure because their safety in this population has not been established.

Hepatic Toxicity

Serum transaminase elevations (2–4). In the phase III trials of troglitazone, 2.2% of patients treated with troglitazone had reversible elevations in AST or ALT greater than three times the upper limit of normal, compared with 0.6% of patients treated with placebo. No evidence of hepatoxicity has been observed with either rosiglitazone or pioglitazone. In the phase III trials of rosiglitazone, 0.2 % of patients treated with rosiglitazone had reversible elevations in ALT greater than three times the upper limit of normal, compared with 0.2% of patients treated with placebo. In the phase III trials of pioglitazone, 0.26% of patients treated with pioglitazone had reversible elevations in ALT greater than three times the upper limit of normal, compared with 0.25% of patients treated with placebo.

Fulminant hepatic failure. Troglitazone was associated with several cases of fulminant hepatic failure resulting in the need for liver transplant or in death (2).

Pregnancy and Nursing

Pioglitazone and rosiglitazone are classified as pregnancy category C (3,4). The currently available thiazolidinediones should not be administered to breast-feeding women (2–4).

SIDE EFFECTS AND MONITORING

Weight Gain

Weight gain appears to be a class effect of the thiazolidinediones.

Pioglitazone. Pioglitazone monotherapy has been associated with a 1.1- to 6.2-lb average weight increase, compared with a 2.86- to 4.18-lb weight loss in patients treated with placebo. In combination with sulfonylureas, pioglitazone has been associated with a 4.2- and 6.4-lb weight gain (15- and 30-mg doses, respectively), compared with a 1.8-lb weight loss in those managed with placebo. Pioglitazone/insulin combination therapy has been associated with a mean 5- and 8.2-lb weight increase (15- and 30-mg doses, respectively), compared with no weight change in placebo-treated patients. Pioglitazone/metformin therapy has been associated with a 2.2-lb weight increase, compared with a 3-lb weight loss in those treated with placebo (4).

Rosiglitazone. Rosiglitazone monotherapy has been associated with a 2.6-lb and 7.7-lb (4- and 8-mg doses, respectively) weight gain. Rosiglitazone/metformin combination therapy has been associated with weight gains of 1.5 and 5 lb (4- and 8-mg doses, respectively). A mean weight loss of 2.2 lb was observed in the placebo and placebo/metformin arms of these studies. Rosiglitazone/sulfonylurea combination therapy was associated with 3.9- and 6.5-lb (4- and 8-mg doses, respectively) weight gains, compared with a 4.3-lb weight gain in patients treated with sulfonylurea alone.

Anemia

Reductions in hemoglobin and hematocrit (≤4% and ≤1 g, respectively) have been observed in patients treated with pioglitazone or rosiglitazone (2–4). These changes are possibly due to volume expansion and have not been associated with significant hematological effects. They occur within the first 4–8 weeks of therapy and have been shown to persist for at least 2 years. These effects are usually mild and no routine monitoring for anemia has been recommended.

Liver Function Abnormalities

Because of the above-mentioned liver function problems associated with troglitazone, routine monthly ALT level measurements were recommended for the first year of therapy and quarterly levels thereafter (2). Currently, it is recommended that patients treated with rosiglitazone or pioglitazone undergo serum transaminase monitoring at the initiation of therapy, every 2 months for the first year, and periodically thereafter (3,4). Additionally, any patient treated with thiazolidinediones who presents with nausea, vomiting, abdominal pain, fatigue, anorexia, or dark urine should have hepatic function tests (2–4). Patients with ALT levels between 1 and 2.5 times the upper limit of normal at baseline or during therapy with pioglitazone or rosiglitazone should be evaluated to determine the cause of the elevation and ALT levels should be monitored frequently (3,4). Patients treated with rosiglitazone or pioglitazone who present with ALT levels greater than or equal to three times the upper limit of normal should have the level rechecked and should discontinue the drug if the elevation persists (3,4).

DRUG INTERACTIONS

Cytochrome P450 enzymes play a role in the metabolism of the thiazolidinediones (2–4). Rosiglitazone is metabolized predominantly by CYP2C8 and to a lesser degree by CYP2C9 (3). In vitro drug metabolism studies have suggested that rosiglitazone does not inhibit the major cytochrome P450 enzymes at clinically relevent concentrations. CYP3A4 is partially responsible for the metabolism of pioglitazone. Studies have also suggested that troglitazone may induce this isoenzyme, which is responsible for the metabolism of several medications including erythromycin, astemizole, calcium-channel antagonists, cisapride, corticosteroids, cyclosporin, HMG-CoA reductase inhibitors, tacrolimus, and some inhibitory drugs, such as ketoconazole and itraconazole. Specific pharmacokinetic studies have not been carried out in many of these agents. The possibility of altered safety and efficacy should always be considered when using the above-mentioned medications with glitazones.

Glyburide

No interaction has been found between glyburide and rosiglitazone (3).

Glipizide

No interaction has been found between glipizide and pioglitazone (4).

Warfarin

No significant effect has been found between warfarin and pioglitazone or rosiglitazone (3,4).

Ethanol

No significant effect has been found between moderate amounts of ethanol and pioglitazone or rosiglitazone (3,4).

Metformin

The pharmacokinetics of metformin when used in combination with rosiglitazone or pioglitazone are unchanged (3,4).

Digoxin

Rosiglitazone and pioglitazone do not alter the pharmacokinetics of digoxin (3–4).

Oral Contraceptives

Administration of troglitazone reduced the serum concentrations of both components of an oral contraceptive containing ethinyl estradiol and norethindrone by 30% (2). Patients taking these two medications may experience a loss of contraception. Pioglitazone has not been evaluated for this possible interaction; therefore, caution should be exercised when using this combination (4). Rosiglitazone has been shown to have no clinically significant effect on the pharmacokinetics of ethinyl estradiol or norethindrone (3).

Ranitidine

Administration of ranitidine did not alter the pharmacokinetics of rosiglitazone, suggesting that the absorption of rosiglitazone is not altered by increases in gastrointestinal pH (3).

Acarbose

Administration of acarbose had no clinically significant effect on the single dose pharmacokinetics of rosiglitazone (3).

Ketoconazole

The administration of ketoconazole in vitro appears to significantly inhibit the metabolism of pioglitazone (4).

CLINICAL EFFECT

Monotherapy

Pioglitazone. In one study, 79 patients with type 2 diabetes (31% drug-naïve, 69% previously treated) were entered into a 26-week trial of monotherapy with pioglitazone (4). Patients were randomized to placebo or 15, 30, or 45 mg pioglitazone after an 8-week washout/run-in period. HbA_{1c} levels in previously naïve patients treated with 15, 30, and 45 mg pioglitazone were 1.4, 1.3, and 2.6% lower, respectively, compared with placebo. HbA_{1c} levels in previously treated patients managed with 15, 30, and 45 mg pioglitazone were 1.0, 0.9, and 1.4% lower, respectively, compared with placebo. Complete glycemic results of that trial are shown in Table 5.3.

In this trial, pioglitazone was associated with 9.0, 9.6, and 9.3% decreases in triglycerides in patients treated with 15, 30, and 45 mg, respectively, compared with baseline. Patients treated with placebo experienced a 4.8% increase in triglycerides. HDL was also altered in this trial. Pioglitazone was associated with 14.1, 12.2, and 19.1% increases in HDL cholesterol in patients treated with 15, 30, and 45 mg, respectively, compared with baseline. Patients treated with placebo experienced an 8.1% increase in HDL. No consistent differences were reported for LDL and total cholesterol in patients treated with pioglitazone versus placebo.

Rosiglitazone. Two 26-week, double-blind, placebo-controlled trials in patients with inadequate glycemic control were carried out with rosiglitazone (4). The results of these studies (A and B) are shown in Tables 5.4 and 5.5. Rosiglitazone was more effective when administered in two divided daily doses than when administered as a single daily dose at the same total daily dosage.

Free fatty acid levels in the monotherapeutic trials were reduced by 7.8 and 14.7% in patients treated with 4 and 8 mg/day, respectively. Patients treated with placebo experienced a 0.2% increase. LDL cholesterol was increased by 14.1 and 18.6% in patients treated with 4 and 8 mg/day, respectively. Patients treated with placebo experienced a 4.8% increase. HDL cholesterol was increased by 11.4 and 14.2% in patients treated with 4 and 8 mg per day, respectively, and patients treated with placebo experienced a 8.0% increase.

Table 5.3 Pioglitazone Monotherapy

	Placebo	Pioglitazone (15 mg/day)	Pioglitazone (30 mg/day)	Pioglitazone (45 mg/day)
Naïve to therapy (*n*)	25	26	26	21
HbA$_{1c}$ (%) (baseline)	9.0	9.9	9.3	10.0
HbA$_{1c}$ (%) (difference from placebo)		−1.4	−1.3	−2.6
FBG (mg/dl) (baseline)	229	251	225	235
FBG (mg/dl) (difference from placebo)		−52	−56	−80
Previously treated (*n*)	54	53	59	55
HbA$_{1c}$ (%) (baseline)	10.9	10.4	10.4	10.6
HbA$_{1c}$ (%) (difference from placebo)		−1.0	−0.9	−1.4
FBG (mg/dl) (baseline)	285	275	286	292
FBG (mg/dl) (difference from placebo)		−36	−31	−59

FBG, fasting blood glucose.

Combination Therapy

Pioglitazone/metformin. A group of 328 patients treated with metformin alone or with metformin and another antidiabetic agent were randomized to either pioglitazone (30 mg/day) or placebo (4). Metformin was continued; however, other antidiabetic agents were discontinued. The addition of pioglitazone to metformin resulted in a mean reduction in HbA$_{1c}$ of 0.8% and a 38 mg/dl (2.1 mmol/l) reduction in fasting blood glucose when compared with placebo. Changes in lipid concentrations were similar to those observed in the monotherapeutic trials.

Rosiglitazone/metformin. Six hundred and seventy patients treated with metformin were evaluated in two prospective, randomized, placebo-controlled combination metformin/rosiglitazone studies (3). In the first

Table 5.4. Rosiglitazone Study A

	Placebo	Rosiglitazone (2 mg bid)	Rosiglitazone (4 mg bid)
n	158	166	169
FPG (mg/dl) (baseline)	229	227	220
FPG (mg/dl) (difference from placebo)		−58	−76
HbA$_{1c}$ (%) (baseline)	9.0	9.0	8.8
HbA$_{1c}$ (%) (difference from placebo)		−1.2	−1.5

trial, metformin (2.5 mg/day) was continued and patients were randomized to receive placebo or 4 or 8 mg/day rosiglitazone. Fasting plasma glucose levels were reduced by 40 mg/dl (2.2 mmol/l) and 53 mg/dl (2.9 mmol/l) in the 4 and 8 mg/day group, respectively, compared with placebo. HbA$_{1c}$ was reduced by 1.0 and 1.2% in the 4 and 8 mg/day groups, respectively, compared with placebo. Changes in LDL and HDL were similar to changes observed in the monotherapy trial.

In a second trial, patients were randomized to combination metformin (2.5 mg/day) and rosiglitazone (4 mg bid) or were discontinued from metformin and started on rosiglitazone monotherapy. Fasting plasma glucose levels were reduced by 56 mg/dl (3.1 mmol/l) in the rosiglitazone/metformin group compared with baseline. HbA$_{1c}$ was reduced by 0.8% in the rosiglitazone/metformin group when compared with baseline. Patients switched to rosiglitazone monotherapy experienced a loss of glycemic control and increases in LDL and VLDL.

Pioglitazone/sulfonylureas. A group of 560 patients treated with sulfonylureas alone or with sulfonylureas and another antidiabetic agent were randomized to either pioglitazone (15 or 30 mg/day) or placebo (4). Sulfonylureas were continued; however, other antidiabetic agents were discontinued. The addition of pioglitazone to sulfonylureas resulted in a mean reduction in HbA$_{1c}$ of 0.9 and 1.3% in the 15 and 30 mg/day groups, respectively. Fasting blood glucose was reduced by 39 and 58 mg/dl (3.2 mmol/l) in the 15 and 30 mg/day groups, respectively. Unfortunately, maximum doses of pioglitazone were not studied. Changes in lipid concentrations were similar to those observed in the monotherapeutic trials.

Pioglitazone/insulin. A group of 566 patients treated with insulin (median dose 60.5 U/day) alone or with another antidiabetic agent were

Table 5.5 Rosiglitazone Study B

	Placebo	Rosiglitazone (4 mg daily)	Rosiglitazone (2 mg bid)	Rosiglitazone (8 mg daily)	Rosiglitazone (4 mg bid)
n	173	180	186	181	187
FPG (mg/dl) (baseline)	225	229	225	228	228
FPG (mg/dl) (difference from placebo)		−31	−43	−49	−62
HbA$_{1c}$ (%) (baseline)	8.9	8.9	8.9	8.9	9.0
HbA$_{1c}$ (%) (difference from placebo)		−0.8	−0.9	−1.1	−1.5

randomized to either pioglitazone (15 or 30 mg/day) or placebo in addition to their insulin (4). Other antidiabetic agents were discontinued. The addition of pioglitazone to insulin resulted in mean reductions in HbA_{1c} of 0.7 and 1.0%, respectively, in the 15 and 30 mg/day groups. Fasting blood glucose was reduced by 35 and 49 mg/dl (1.9 and 2.7 mmol/l), respectively, in the 15 and 30 mg/day groups. Unfortunately, maximum doses of pioglitazone were not studied. Changes in lipid concentrations were similar to those observed in the monotherapeutic trials.

REFERENCES

1. Henry RR: Thiazolidinediones: current therapies for diabetes. *Endocrinol Metab Clin North Am* 26:553–573, 1997

2. Rezulin (troglitazone) package insert, Parke-Davis, 1999

3. Avandia (rosiglitazone) package insert, SmithKline Beecham, 1999

4. Actos (pioglitazone) package insert, Eli Lilly, 1999

5. Ehrmann DA, Schneider DJ, Sobel BE, Cavaghan MK, Imperial J, Rosenfield RL, Polansky KS: Troglitazone improves defects in insulin action, insulin secretion, ovarian steroidogenesis and fibrinolysis in women with polycystic ovarian syndrome. *J Clin Endocrinol Metab* 82:2108–2116, 1997

6. White J: The pharmacologic reduction of blood glucose in patients with type 2 diabetes mellitus. *Clin Diabetes* 16:58–67, 1998

7. Saleh YM, Mudaliar SR, Henry RR: Metabolic and vascular effects of the thiazolidinedione troglitazone. *Diabetes Rev* 7:55–76, 1999

8. Saltiel AR, Olefsky JM: Thiazolidinediones in the treatment of insulin resistance and type II diabetes. *Diabetes* 45:1661–1669, 1996

6. Meglitinide Products

Quick Reference

Mechanism of Action: The only meglitinide product currently available in the U.S. for the treatment of diabetes is repaglinide (Prandin, NovoNordisk). It is structurally unrelated to the sulfonylureas, but like that therapeutic class, lowers blood glucose levels by stimulating insulin release from the pancreas. Repaglinide has a more rapid onset of action and a shorter duration of action than the sulfonylureas.

Pharmacokinetics: Repaglinide is rapidly absorbed following oral administration. Administration with food lowers the amount of drug absorbed. The drug is metabolized by the cytochrome P450 3A4 isoenzymes of the liver to inactive metabolites. The elimination half-life of repaglinide is 1 h. This may be shortened by enzyme inducers or increased by enzyme inhibitors.

Dosage Forms and Dose: The initial starting dose of repaglinide is 0.5 mg if the patient is naïve to treatment or if the patient's HbA_{1c} is <8%. The initial dose is 1 or 2 mg before each meal for patients who have previously been treated with blood glucose–lowering drugs and whose HbA_{1c} is ≥8%. The maximum daily dose is 16 mg. Repaglinide is available in 0.5-, 1-, and 2-mg tablets.

Special Populations: Repaglinide should be used with caution in patients with moderate to severe liver dysfunction.

Precautions and Side Effects: Repaglinide is contraindicated in patients with diabetic ketoacidosis, type 1 diabetes, or known hypersensitivity to repaglinide or any of the product's ingredients. The most commonly reported adverse effects include hypoglycemia, upper respiratory infections, sinusitis, nausea, diarrhea, constipation, arthralgia, and headache. Hypoglycemia may occur more frequently in patients with hepatic, adrenal, or pituitary insufficiency, as well as in elderly, debilitated, or malnourished patients.

INTRODUCTION

The meglitinide agents were developed to be structurally and pharmacologically unrelated to the sulfonylureas. These agents were designed to promote an insulin release profile similar to physiological glucose-stimulated insulin release. The meglitinide agents are intended to be taken only when the patient eats, thus allowing the patient more freedom in the timing of meals. They were also designed to have a short half-life to reduce the risk of hypoglycemia.

PHARMACOLOGY

Mechanism of Action

Repaglinide (Prandin) is a meglitinide blood glucose–lowering agent. The meglitinide class is structurally unrelated to the sulfonylureas, but like that class, lowers blood glucose levels by stimulating insulin release from the pancreas. As with the sulfonylureas, release of insulin is dependent on functioning β-cells in the pancreatic islets; it is glucose dependent and diminishes at low glucose concentrations. Also like the sulfonylureas, repaglinide closes ATP-dependent potassium channels in the pancreatic islet β-cell membrane. Potassium channel blockade depolarizes the β-cell, which leads to an opening of calcium channels; this results in an increased calcium influx, which induces insulin secretion (1–7). Repaglinide has a more rapid onset and a shorter duration of action than the sulfonylureas.

Pharmacokinetics

Peak plasma concentrations of repaglinide are reached within 1 h following oral administration. The mean absolute bioavailability is 56%. Administration with food does not affect the time to peak, but it reduces the mean peak concentration by 20% and the area under the plasma time concentration curve (AUC) is reduced by 12.4% (1). The volume of distribution is 31 liters, and protein binding is >98% (1).

The elimination half-life is ~1 h (1). Repaglinide is metabolized via oxidative biotransformation and conjugation to inactive metabolites (1,8). The metabolites are primarily excreted in the feces (90%) (1,8). Only 0.1% of the repaglinide dose is excreted unchanged in the urine, and <2% is excreted unchanged in the feces (1).

INDICATIONS

Repaglinide is indicated as an adjunct to nutrition and exercise to lower blood glucose in patients with type 2 diabetes whose hyperglycemia cannot be controlled satisfactorily by nutrition and exercise alone. It is also indicated for use in combination with metformin to lower blood glucose in patients whose hyperglycemia cannot be controlled by exercise, nutrition, and either repaglinide or metformin alone (1).

DOSING CONSIDERATIONS

Dosage Forms

Repaglinide is available in 0.5-, 1-, and 2-mg tablets. Repaglinide should be stored at controlled room temperature (<25°C) and protected from moisture (1).

Dosage and Administration

For patients not previously treated or whose HbA_{1c} is <8%, the starting dose should be 0.5 mg. For patients previously treated with blood glucose–lowering drugs and whose HbA_{1c} is ≥8%, the initial dose is 1 or 2 mg before each meal (1). Dosage adjustments should be determined by blood glucose response. The preprandial dose should be increased until satisfactory blood glucose control is achieved or until a maximum dose of 4 mg/dose or 16 mg/day is reached. Most dosage adjustments should be done at weekly intervals or longer, but dosage adjustments in patients with hepatic insufficiency should be less frequent (1).

Glycemic control has been shown to be maintained with administration before meals when two, three, or four meals per day are eaten (corresponding to two, three, or four doses per day) and repaglinide is administered at the start of the meal or 15 or 30 min before the meal (1). Doses are usually taken within 15 min of the meal, but may be taken any time from immediately before to as long as 30 min before the meal (1). Patients who skip a meal or add an extra meal should be instructed to skip or add a dose for that meal, respectively (1,9).

When repaglinide replaces another oral hypoglycemic agent, the first repaglinide dose may be administered on the day after the final dose of the other agent is given. After conversion to repaglinide, patients should be monitored closely for hypoglycemia. In particular, when a patient is switched from a sulfonylurea with a longer half-life, close monitoring for up to 1 week or longer may be indicated (1).

Metformin may be administered concomitantly with repaglinide therapy in patients not adequately controlled on either agent alone. The starting repaglinide dosage is the same as for monotherapy (1,10).

SPECIAL POPULATIONS

Renal Dysfunction

Patients with renal dysfunction may have increased AUC and peak serum repaglinide levels. No adjustment in the initial dose of repaglinide is necessary (1).

Hepatic Dysfunction

Patients with moderate to severe impairment of liver function will have higher serum concentrations and more unbound repaglinide and metabolites than will patients with normal hepatic function. However, the altered serum concentrations and unbound fraction have not been shown to alter the response to the repaglinide. It may be possible that some patients with hepatic dysfunction will respond differently and may require longer dosing intervals and/or lower doses of repaglinide (1).

Geriatrics

The pharmacokinetics of repaglinide are not affected by age (1).

Pediatrics

Repaglinide is not indicated for the treatment of infants and children. The safety and effectiveness of repaglinide have not been established in this patient population (1).

Ethnic Groups

Ethnicity does not appear to affect the pharmacokinetics of repaglinide (1).

Sex

Women may have a higher AUC (15–70%), but the frequency of adverse events or hypoglycemia is not increased. Adjustments in dose should be based on clinical response and not on sex (1).

CONTRAINDICATIONS

Repaglinide is contraindicated in patients with diabetic ketoacidosis, type 1 diabetes, or known hypersensitivity to repaglinide or any of the product's inactive ingredients (calcium hydrogen phosphate, microcrystalline cellulose, maize starch, polacrilin potassium, povidone, glycerol, magnesium stearate, meglumine, poloxamer, and iron oxide dyes) (1).

PRECAUTIONS

Periodic monitoring of fasting blood glucose and HbA_{1c} levels is recommended. During dosage adjustment, fasting blood glucose can be used to determine therapeutic response. Thereafter, both glucose and HbA_{1c} should be monitored. Monitoring of HbA_{1c} every 3 months is recommended (1).

A warning regarding increased risk of cardiovascular mortality with oral hypoglycemic drugs is included in the product label. This is a warning that is required in the labeling of oral hypoglycemic drugs based on the University Group Diabetes Program study that was published in 1970 (1). This increased risk has not been documented with repaglinide, but is a required part of its labeling.

Hypoglycemia

Repaglinide is capable of producing hypoglycemia. Patients with hepatic, adrenal, or pituitary insufficiency, as well as elderly, debilitated, or malnourished patients, may be more susceptible (1). In comparative trials with glyburide and glipizide, hypoglycemia was reported in 16% of repaglinide-treated patients, 20% of glyburide-treated patients, and 19% of glipizide-treated patients (1). The frequency of hypoglycemia is greatest in patients who have not been previously treated with oral blood glucose–lowering agents and those with an HbA_{1c} <8% (1). The risk of hypoglycemia is lessened by administering the repaglinide dose with food (1).

Loss of Control of Blood Glucose

If the patient experiences stress, such as fever, trauma, infection, or surgery, it may be necessary to replace the repaglinide with insulin therapy (1).

Long-term therapy may be associated with a decrease in glycemic control. If this happens, the patient's adherence to nutrition therapy should be assessed and an adjustment in dose considered. However, if adherence to nutrition therapy is good and the dose of repaglinide has been maximized, this could be classified as a secondary failure (1).

Pregnancy and Nursing

Repaglinide is categorized in pregnancy category C (1). Repaglinide was not teratogenic in animal studies. However, nonteratogenic skeletal deformities were observed following exposure during gestation and lactation. Abnormal blood glucose levels during pregnancy are associated with a higher incidence of congenital abnormalities; therefore, insulin therapy is recommended during pregnancy to maintain blood glucose levels as close to normal as possible (1).

The manufacturer recommends that repaglinide not be administered to nursing mothers. It is not known if repaglinide is excreted in human milk, but it is in some animals. This recommendation is based on the risk of hypoglycemia and the concern that skeletal deformities, such as those observed in the animal studies, may occur (1).

Pediatrics

The safety and effectiveness of repaglinide have not been established in children. However, repaglinide is contraindicated in the care of type 1 diabetes (1).

SIDE EFFECTS AND MONITORING

The adverse effects most commonly reported during repaglinide therapy have included hypoglycemia, upper respiratory infections, sinusitis, nausea, diarrhea, constipation, arthralgia, weight gain, and headache (see Table 6.1) (1). Monitoring blood glucose levels and only taking repaglinide if a meal is to be consumed can help to reduce the risk of hypoglycemia. Paying closer attention to nutrition, consuming fewer calories, and exercising more can help to prevent the weight gain.

DRUG INTERACTIONS

Repaglinide metabolism may be inhibited by inhibitors of CYP 3A4, such as ketoconazole, miconazole, and erythromycin. Agents that induce CYP 3A4 metabolism, such as troglitazone, rifampin, barbiturates, and carbamazepine, may reduce repaglinide levels (1). Phase IV studies evaluating the potential for interactions between repaglinide and HMG-CoA reductase inhibitors, estrogen, and calcium channel blockers are in progress (11).

Table 6.1 Percentage of Patients Commonly Reporting Adverse Effects of Repaglinide

Adverse Effect	Placebo-Controlled Studies		Active-Controlled Studies	
	Repaglinide (*n* = 352)	Placebo (*n* = 108)	Repaglinide (*n* = 1228)	Sulfonylurea (*n* = 498)
Arthralgia	6	3	3	4
Back pain	5	4	6	7
Bronchitis	2	1	6	7
Constipation	3	2	2	3
Diarrhea	5	2	4	6
Dyspepsia	2	2	4	2
Headache	11	10	9	8
Hypoglycemia	31	7	16	20
Nausea	5	5	3	2
Paresthesia	3	3	2	1
Rhinitis	3	3	7	8
Sinusitis	6	2	3	4
Upper respiratory tract infection	16	8	10	10
Vomiting	3	3	2	1

From the package insert (1).

Repaglinide does not interact with digoxin, theophylline, warfarin, or cimetidine (1,12).

The hypoglycemic action of repaglinide may be potentiated by nonsteroidal anti-inflammatory drugs (NSAIDs) and other agents that are highly plasma-protein bound, salicylates, sulfonamides, chloramphenicol, coumarins, probenecid, monoamine oxidase inhibitors, troglitazone, and β-blockers (1,13). Loss of glycemic control may occur with concomitant administration with agents that may produce hyperglycemia, such as thiazides and other diuretics, corticosteroids, phenothiazines, thyroid products, estrogens, oral contraceptives, phenytoin, nicotinic acid, sympathomimetics, calcium channel blockers, and isoniazid (1).

CLINICAL EFFECT

The results of several studies are summarized in the repaglinide package insert. In one 4-week, double-blind, placebo-controlled study enrolling 138 patients with type 2 diabetes, repaglinide doses of 0.25–4.00 mg taken with each meal were evaluated. Dose-proportional reductions in glucose were observed over this dosage range. Insulin levels increased after meals, then reverted toward baseline before the next meal. Effects were apparent within 1–2 weeks (1).

In another double-blind, placebo-controlled study, repaglinide doses were titrated weekly over a range of 0.25–4 mg, until a fasting plasma glucose level of <160 mg/dl (8.88 mmol/l) was achieved or the 4-mg maximum dose was reached. Fasting plasma glucose and 2-h postprandial glucose increased in the placebo-treated patients and decreased in the repaglinide-treated patients. Fasting plasma glucose was 61 mg/dl (3.39 mmol/l) lower in the repaglinide group compared with that in the placebo group, while postprandial glucose was 104 mg/dl (5.77 mmol/l) lower in the repaglinide group than in the placebo group. HbA$_{1c}$ was 1.7% units lower in the repaglinide group. Results are summarized in Figures 6.1 and 6.2 (1).

In another double-blind, placebo-controlled study enrolling 362 patients, 1- and 4-mg preprandial doses of repaglinide were shown to reduce fasting blood glucose and HbA$_{1c}$ compared with placebo. In patients who had not previously been treated, the HbA$_{1c}$ was reduced by 2.1% in the repaglinide groups compared with the placebo group. In patients previously treated with a sulfonylurea, HbA$_{1c}$ was reduced by 1.7% in the repaglinide group compared with the placebo group. Blood glucose–lowering effects, including hypoglycemia, were most apparent in patients who were naïve to oral-hypoglycemic-agent therapy

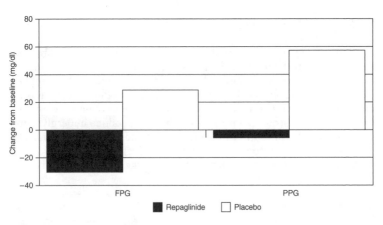

Figure 6.1 Effects on glucose parameters after 3 months of repaglinide and placebo in patients with type 2 diabetes. From the package insert for Prandin (1). FPG, fasting plasma glucose; PPG, postprandial glucose.

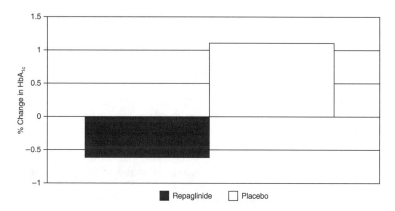

Figure 6.2 Effects on HbA$_{1c}$ after 3 months of repaglinide and placebo in patients with type 2 diabetes. From the package insert for Prandin (1).

and who were in relatively good glycemic control before therapy (HbA$_{1c}$ <8%). Weight gain was not observed in patients previously treated with oral hypoglycemic agents; however, in patients naïve to oral-hypoglycemic-agent therapy, the average weight gain in the repaglinide group was 3.3% (1).

In another small study (n = 18), administration of repaglinide three times daily before meals was more effective than administration twice daily before the morning and evening meal. Fasting blood glucose was reduced in both treatment groups; however, glycemic control, as demonstrated by reductions in HbA$_{1c}$, was achieved only in the group receiving repaglinide three times daily (14).

The efficacy of repaglinide is comparable to that of glyburide and glicazide and greater than that of glipizide (11,15). In a study enrolling 44 patients with type 2 diabetes, repaglinide and glyburide demonstrated similar effects. Patients received either repaglinide (1–4 mg/day) or glyburide (10–15 mg/day) twice daily for 12 weeks. Doses were taken 15 min before the morning and evening meals. Glyburide reduced fasting blood glucose with no effect on postprandial blood glucose. Repaglinide reduced postprandial blood glucose with no effect on fasting blood glucose. Glycated hemoglobin was unchanged in both groups. Fasting plasma insulin was reduced in the repaglinide group, but not in the glyburide group (16).

In another study, repaglinide and glyburide were compared in 195 patients with type 2 diabetes. Patients were treated with 0.5, 1, 2, or 4 mg repaglinide before the three main meals or with 1.75, 3.5, 7, or

10.5 mg glyburide administered in the morning or in divided doses twice daily for 14 weeks. HbA$_{1c}$ and fasting blood glucose were reduced to a similar extent in both treatment groups. Mean blood glucose and 2-h postbreakfast blood glucose were lower in the repaglinide group. The frequencies of hypoglycemic episodes were comparable (17–19). Similar results have been reported by other investigators (20).

Combination repaglinide and metformin therapy has been evaluated in a study enrolling 83 patients whose blood glucose was not controlled by exercise, nutrition, and metformin alone. Patients were treated with metformin (1–3 g/day), repaglinide (0.5–4 mg) three times daily before meals, or a combination of the two. Synergistic improvement in glycemic control compared with repaglinide and metformin monotherapy was observed. HbA$_{1c}$ was improved by 1%, and fasting plasma glucose was reduced by an additional 35 mg/dl (1.94 mmol/l). Results of this study are summarized in Table 6.2. More gastrointestinal side effects were observed in the patients treated with metformin or metformin plus repaglinide (1,10,21,22).

The combination of NPH insulin and repaglinide may improve glycemic control in patients with type 2 diabetes who are inadequately controlled with sulfonylurea or sulfonylurea plus metformin. In one study, the addition of NPH insulin to repaglinide therapy did not increase the risk of serious hypoglycemia, but it did increase the number of mild hypoglycemic episodes (23,24).

PATIENT COUNSELING

Adherence to nutrition therapy and an exercise program is necessary to get the maximum benefit from repaglinide therapy. Patients should be encouraged to test their blood glucose on a regular basis and to report

Table 6.2 Combined Repaglinide and Metformin Therapy

	Repaglinide	Combination	Metformin
Number of patients	28	27	27
HbA$_{1c}$ (%) (change from baseline)	–0.38	–1.41	–0.33
Fasting plasma glucose (mg/dl [mmol/l]) (change from baseline)	8.8 [0.49]	–39.2 [–2.18]	–4.5 [–0.25]

From the package insert and Moses and colleagues (21,22).

variations and increases to their primary care giver. Changes in lifestyle or stresses, such as fever, trauma, infection, or surgery, may alter glucose control and necessitate a change in therapy.

Patients should also be taught the signs and symptoms of hypoglycemia and what to do if hypoglycemia should occur.

REFERENCES

1. Prandin (repaglinide) package insert, NovoNordisk, 1997

2. Malaisse WJ: Insulinotropic action of meglitinide analogues: modulation by an activator of ATP-sensitive K^+ channels and high extracellular K^+ concentrations. *Pharmacol Res* 32:111–114, 1995

3. Jijakli H, Ulusoy S, Malaisse WJ: Dissociation between the potency and reversibility of the insulinotropic action of two meglitinide analogues. *Pharmacol Res* 34:105–108, 1996

4. Malaisse WJ: Stimulation of insulin release by non-sulfonylurea hypoglycemic agents: the meglitinide family. *Horm Metab Res* 27:263–266, 1995

5. Gromada J, Dissing S, Kofod H, Frokjaer-Jensen J: Effects of the hypoglycaemic drugs repaglinide and glibenclamide on ATP-sensitive potassium-channels and cytosolic calcium levels in β TC3 cells and rat pancreatic beta cells. *Diabetologia* 38:1025–1032, 1995

6. Melander A: Oral antidiabetic drugs: an overview. *Diabetic Med* 13:S143–S147, 1996

7. Fuhlendorff J, Rorsman P, Kofod H, Brand CL, Rolin B, MacKay P, Shymko R, Carr RD: Stimulation of insulin release by repaglinide and glibenclamide involves both common and distinct processes. *Diabetes* 47:345–351, 1998

8. Bauer E, Beschke K, Ebner T, Greischel A, Heinle R, Prox A, Schiller-Rankewitz H, Schmid J, Stangier J, Wachsmuth H, Wolfinger H: Biotransformation of [14C]repaglinide in human, cynomolgus monkey, dog, rabbit, rat and mouse (Abstract). *Diabetologia* 40 (Suppl. 1):A326, 1997

9. Hatorp V, Marbury TC, Damsbo P, Gawrylewski H: Repaglinide can be given in a flexible preprandial dosing regimen to patients with type II diabetes (Abstract). *Diabetes* 46 (Suppl. 1):151A, 1997

10. Moses R, Slobodniuk R, Boyages S, Colagiuri S, Kidson W, Carter J, Donnelly T, Moffitt P, Hopkins H: Effect of repaglinide addition to metformin monotherapy on glycemic control in patients with type 2 diabetes. *Diabetes Care* 22:119–124, 1999

11. Anon.: Novo Nordisk Prandin to be launched in spring 1998; drug interaction with statins, estrogen, calcium channel blockers to be evaluated as part of Phase IV commitments. *Health News Daily*, F-D-C Reports, Inc. 1997;9(248):1

12. Strange P, Rosenberg MA, Cohen A: Assessment of pharmacokinetic (PK) and pharmacodynamic (PD) interaction between warfarin and repaglinide (Abstract). *Diabetes* 48 (Suppl. 1):A356, 1999

13. Raskin P, Kennedy F, Woo V, Jain R, Boss AH: A multicenter, randomized study of the therapeutic effect of repaglinide combined with troglitazone in subjects with type 2 diabetes. *Diabetes* 48 (Suppl. 1):A107, 1999

14. Damsbo P, Andersen PH, Lund S, Porksen N: Improved glycaemic control with repaglinide in NIDDM with 3 times daily meal related dosing (Abstract). *Diabetes* 46 (Suppl. 1):34A, 1997

15. Anon.: Novo Prandin for type 2 diabetes may reduce hypoglycemia—FDA's Fleming; pre-prandial dosing regimen and rapid action differentiate Prandin. *The Pink Sheet*, F-D-C Reports, Inc. 1997;59(47):3

16. Wolffenbuttel BHR, Nijst L, Sels JPJE, Menheere PPCA, Muller PG, Nieuwenhuijzen Kruseman AC: Effects of a new oral hypoglycaemic agent, repaglinide, on metabolic control in sulphonylurea-treated patients with NIDDM. *Eur J Clin Pharmacol* 45:113–116, 1993

17. Landgraf R, Bilo HJG: Repaglinide vs glibenclamide: a 14-week efficacy and safety comparison (Abstract). *Diabetes* 46 (Suppl. 1):162A, 1997

18. Landgraf R, Bilo HJG: Repaglinide vs glibenclamide: a 14-week efficacy and safety comparison (Abstract). *Diabetologia* 40 (Suppl. 1):A321, 1997

19. Landgraf R, Bilo HJ, Muller PG: A comparison of repaglinide and glibenclamide in the treatment of type 2 diabetic patients previously treated with sulphonylureas. *Eur J Clin Pharmacol* 55:165–171, 1999

20. Wolffenbuttel BH, Landgraf R, Dutch and German Repaglinide Study Group: A 1-year multicenter randomized double-blind com-

parison of repaglinide and glyburide for the treatment of type 2 diabetes. *Diabetes Care* 22:463–467, 1999

21. Moses R, Slobodniuk R, Boyages S, Colagiuri S, Kidson W, Carter J, Donnelly T, Moffitt P, Hopkins H: Additional treatment with repaglinide provides significant improvement in glycaemic control in NIDDM patients poorly controlled on metformin (Abstract). *Diabetologia* 40 (Suppl. 1):A322, 1997

22. Moses R, Slododniuk R, Donnelly T, Moffitt P, Boyages S, Colagiuri S, Kidson W, Carter J: Additional treatment with repaglinide provides significant improvement in glycaemic control in NIDDM patients poorly controlled on metformin (Abstract). *Diabetes* 46 (Suppl. 1):93A, 1997

23. Landin-Olsson M, Brogard JMM, Eriksson J, Rasmussen M, Clauson P: The efficacy of repaglinide administered in combination with bedtime NPH-insulin in patients with type 2 diabetes: a randomized, semi-blinded, parallel-group, multi-centre trial (Abstract). *Diabetes* 48 (Suppl. 1):A117, 1999

24. Eriksson JG, Brogard JM, Landin-Olsson M, Clauson P, Rasmussen M: The safety of repaglinide administered in combination with bedtime NPH-insulin in patients with type 2 diabetes: a randomized, semi-blinded, parallel-group, multi-centre trial. *Diabetes* 48 (Suppl. 1):A360, 1999

7. Biguanides

Quick Reference

Biguanides: Only one biguanide is currently available in the U.S.: metformin (Glucophage, Bristol-Myers Squibb).

Mechanism of Action: Although metformin causes a number of metabolic effects, including changes in carbohydrate, lipid, and protein metabolism, the primary effect is on carbohydrate metabolism, lowering blood glucose levels by reducing insulin resistance.

Pharmacokinetics: Metformin is fairly well absorbed, with an absolute bioavailability of between 50 and 60%. The drug is eliminated completely unchanged via the urine. Although food does not significantly alter the bioavailability of metformin, metformin is normally administered just before meals to reduce side effects.

Dosage Forms and Dose: Metformin hydrochloride is available in 500- or 850-mg tablets. The usual starting dose of metformin is 500 mg twice daily given with the morning and evening meals. Doses may be titrated up to as high as 2,550 mg and may be given as often as three times a day.

Special Populations: Metformin should be avoided in patients with renal or hepatic insufficiency. Limited data are available in the geriatric population, and no data are available in the pediatric population.

Precautions and Side Effects: Metformin should be used only in patients with good renal function, and renal function should be monitored periodically. Metformin should be discontinued in patients requiring studies with iodinated contrast media. It should be avoided in patients with medical conditions leading to hypoxic states, such as cardiovascular collapse, acute congestive heart failure, or acute myocardial infarction. Additionally, metformin should be temporarily discontinued in any patient undergoing a major surgical procedure. Patients with significant alcohol intake or patients with impaired hepatic function should not be treated with metformin. Primary side effects include gastrointestinal symptoms, such as abdominal bloating, flatulence, anorexia, diarrhea, nausea, and vomiting. Lactic acidosis occurs rarely.

INTRODUCTION

The historical beginning of the biguanides is in medieval times, when French lilac, or goat's rue, (*galega officinalis*) was used as a folk treatment for diabetes in southern and eastern Europe (1). Later, *g. officinalis* was found to be rich in the compound guanidine. In 1918, the hypoglycemic activity of guanidine was confirmed (1). Unfortunately, guanidine was too toxic for human clinical use, but its chemical congeners, such as the alkyldiguanide SynthalinA, were introduced in the early 1920s. Further analysis continued with the biguanide group in the 1920s (1); however, clinical use of these compounds was not pursued. The compounds fell into disfavor because of the discovery and availability of insulin products.

With the advent of sulfonylureas in the 1950s, biguanides were reinvestigated for possible use in the treatment of diabetes. Metformin and phenformin were introduced in 1957, followed by buformin in 1958 (1). No other active compounds in the biguanide category have been discovered, even though significant work on the structure-activity relationship has taken place. Clinical use of buformin was limited, but phenformin was used widely in the 1960s and 1970s. An association between phenformin and lactic acidosis resulted in the withdrawal of this compound from use in many countries. Recently, metformin has become the most relevant drug of the biguanide category. It was approved for use in the U.S. in the 1990s (2).

PHARMACOLOGY

Mechanism of Action

Metformin causes a plethora of metabolic effects including changes in carbohydrate, lipid, and lipoprotein metabolism (3). The primary effect of metformin on carbohydrate metabolism is via its effects on insulin resistance. The effects of metformin on carbohydrate metabolism occur primarily at the liver. Metformin's main effect is associated with a reduction in basal hepatic glucose output in patients with type 2 diabetes. This reduction is responsible for a significant mechanism of action by which metformin reduces blood glucose levels (4). Numerous studies have shown metformin's effect on hepatic glucose production in patients with type 2 diabetes. Whereas one study suggested that this effect was mediated via a reduction in glycogenolysis, another study concluded that the effect may be secondary to a reduction in gluconeogenesis (5,6).

Metformin also has been shown to lower blood glucose by enhancing insulin-stimulated glucose transport in skeletal muscle. The observed enhancement of glucose uptake ranges from 10 to 40% depending on the population being studied (7); however, this may be indirect, due to improvement of glucose toxicity (8). Lastly, metformin decreases fatty acid oxidation by as much as 20%, which causes a reduction in plasma glucose concentrations by changes in the glucose fatty acid cycle (4).

Pharmacokinetics

The absolute bioavailability of metformin ranges from 50 to 60%. The compound is absorbed mainly from the small intestine, with an estimated absorption half-life of between 0.09 and 2.6 h. The maximum concentration (C_{max}) of 1–2 μg/ml is reached ~1–2 h after an oral dose of between 500 and 1,000 mg. The drug undergoes negligible binding to plasma proteins. The half-life of metformin in individuals with normal renal function ranges from 1.5 to 4.9 h (4). No measurable metabolism of metformin occurs.

In terms of elimination, ~90% of the compound is excreted via the urine within 12 h of administration of the dose. The elimination of the drug occurs via glomerular filtration and tubular secretion. Tubular secretion is thought to be a major route of metformin elimination because the renal clearance of this compound is ~3.5 times greater than creatinine clearance (9). The drug is widely distributed into most tissues in concentrations similar to those found in peripheral plasma. However, the highest concentrations are found in the salivary glands and in the intestinal wall. Relatively high concentrations are found in the liver and the kidney (4).

Indications

Metformin hydrochloride is indicated for monotherapeutic management of type 2 diabetes as an adjunct to nutrition and exercise in patients whose hyperglycemia cannot be satisfactorily managed by nutrition therapy alone. Additionally, metformin may be used concomitantly with a sulfonylurea when nutrition and metformin therapy or sulfonylurea and nutrition therapy do not result in adequate glycemic control (9). Metformin is also approved for use with pioglitazone (10), rosiglitazone (11), and repaglinide (12).

DOSING CONSIDERATIONS

Dosage Forms

Metformin hydrochloride is available in 500- and 850-mg tablets (9).

Dosage and Administration

The usual starting dose is two 500-mg metformin tablets, one taken with the morning meal and one with the evening meal. Doses may be titrated in increments of one tablet every week up to a maximum of 2,550 mg per day. Metformin is often administered at a dose of 1,000 mg twice a day with the morning and evening meals. If a dose of 2,550 mg is required, the patient may tolerate it better if it is given three times a day with meals.

The usual starting dose of 850-mg metformin tablets is once daily, given with the morning meal. Dosage increases are usually made in increments of one tablet every other week given in divided doses up to a maximum of 2,550 mg per day. The most common maintenance dose is 850 mg given twice a day with the morning and evening meals. However, if necessary, patients may be given 850 mg three times a day with meals.

SPECIAL POPULATIONS

Renal Insufficiency

In patients with reduced renal function, the plasma half-life of metformin is prolonged and the renal clearance is reduced in proportion to the decrease in creatinine clearance (9). For example, the renal clearance of metformin in a healthy nondiabetic patient with normal renal function given a dose of 850 mg is 552 ml/min, in comparison with patients with mildly (creatinine clearance 61–90 ml/min), moderately (creatinine clearance 31–60 ml/min), or severely (creatinine clearance 10–30 ml/min) impaired renal function, who demonstrate metformin clearances of 384, 108, and 130 ml/min, respectively (9).

Hepatic Insufficiency

No pharmacokinetic data are available in patients with hepatic insufficiency.

Geriatrics

Limited data are available from controlled pharmacokinetic studies evaluating the effects of age on metformin kinetics. However, it is known that total plasma clearance is lower, half-life is longer, and C_{max} is higher than in healthy young subjects. It appears that the change in metformin pharmacokinetics with aging is secondary to the changes in renal function that occur in the geriatric population.

Pediatrics

No pharmacokinetic data are available in pediatric patients.

Sex

No pharmacokinetic differences have been observed between the sexes. Clinically, in controlled trials in patients with type 2 diabetes, no differences have been observed between male and female patients.

Ethnicity

Although no pharmacokinetic studies have been carried out evaluating differences between ethnic groups in controlled clinical trials, the effects of metformin have been shown to be comparable in non-Hispanic white, black, and Hispanic subjects (9).

CONTRAINDICATIONS

Metformin is contraindicated in patients with

- acute or chronic metabolic acidosis
- known hypersensitivity to metformin hydrochloride
- congestive heart failure requiring pharmacological management
- renal disease or dysfunction (serum creatinine levels ≥1.5 mg/dl in male or ≥1.4 mg/dl in female patients) or abnormal creatinine clearance that may result from medical conditions such as cardiovascular collapse, acute myocardial infarction, or septicemia
- age >80 years, unless measurement of creatinine clearance demonstrates adequate renal function

Metformin should be discontinued temporarily in patients requiring radiological studies involving the use of iodinated contrast media because these agents are known to cause renal dysfunction in some individuals.

PRECAUTIONS

Monitoring Renal Function

Metformin is known to be excreted via the kidneys; thus, the risk of accumulation of the medication is greater in patients with reduced renal function. The risk of lactic acidosis is increased in these patients as well. Therefore, patients with serum creatinine levels above the upper limit of normal for their age should not be treated with metformin (9). In elderly patients, renal function should be monitored periodically. This medication should not be used in patients >80 years of age unless measurement of creatinine clearance demonstrates that renal function is not reduced. It should be noted that these patients are more susceptible to the development of lactic acidosis.

Radiological Studies

Radiological studies involving the use of iodinated contrast media should be undertaken only after metformin has been discontinued. The drug should be withheld for at least 48 h after the procedure and reinstituted only after serum creatinine levels have been shown to be normal (9).

Hypoxic States

Lactic acidosis is associated with cardiovascular collapse, acute congestive heart failure, acute myocardial infarction, and other conditions that cause hypoxemia. Therefore, metformin should be discontinued in patients with these medical conditions.

Surgical Procedures

Metformin therapy should be discontinued temporarily for any major surgical procedure and should be restarted only after the patient's oral intake has been resumed and renal function has been shown to be normal (9).

Alcohol Intake

Metformin should be used cautiously in patients who are known to consume excessive alcohol, since this may lead to acidosis.

Impaired Hepatic Function

Impaired hepatic function has been associated with some cases of lactic acidosis; therefore, it is recommended that metformin not be used in patients with impaired hepatic function.

Vitamin B$_{12}$ Levels

Seven percent of patients who are treated with metformin experience a reduction in vitamin B$_{12}$ to subnormal levels. However, this is rarely associated with anemia and appears to be rapidly reversible with discontinuation of the medication or with vitamin B$_{12}$ supplementation. Patients treated with metformin should therefore undergo measurement of hematological parameters annually. Hematological evaluation is also advised in any patient with apparent abnormalities. Routine serum vitamin B$_{12}$ measurements approximately every 2–3 years may be useful in individuals with inadequate B$_{12}$ or calcium intake and/or absorption.

Hypoglycemia

Hypoglycemia does not occur with metformin monotherapy under normal conditions. However, it may occur in patients in whom caloric intake is deficient, in patients who undertake strenuous exercise, in patients who are treated with other glucose-lowering agents, such as sulfonylureas, or in patients who consume ethanol (9).

SIDE EFFECTS AND MONITORING

Lactic Acidosis

Lactic acidosis is a very rare but extremely serious condition that can occur secondary to the accumulation of metformin (9). Lactic acidosis is fatal in ~50% of cases. Currently, the reported incidence of lactic acidosis in patients receiving metformin is extremely low, ~0.03 cases per 1,000 patient-years, with a fatality rate of ~0.015 fatal cases per 1,000 patient-years. The majority of these cases have occurred in patients with significant renal insufficiency. The risk of lactic acidosis can be reduced by observing the aforementioned contraindications and precautions.

Gastrointestinal Reactions

Gastrointestinal symptoms, such as abdominal bloating, flatulence, anorexia, diarrhea, nausea, and vomiting, are the most common side effects observed in patients treated with metformin. Gastrointestinal complaints are ~30% more frequent in patients on metformin monotherapy than in patients treated with placebo, particularly during the initial phases of therapy. These complaints are generally transient and may resolve with continued treatment. In some cases, however, temporary dose reduction may be prudent (9). Gastrointestinal symptoms during initial therapy may be mitigated if patients are treated via gradual dose escalation and counseled to take their medication with meals. If significant diarrhea and/or vomiting occur, metformin should be temporarily discontinued.

Dysgeusia

Approximately 3% of patients treated with metformin will complain of an unpleasant or metallic taste in their mouths. This usually resolves spontaneously.

Dermatological Reactions

In controlled trials, the incidence of rash or dermatitis in patients treated with metformin monotherapy was comparable to that with placebo.

Hematological Reactions

As mentioned above, metformin therapy may result in a small reduction in vitamin B_{12} levels; however, only five cases of megaloblastic anemia have been reported with metformin administration worldwide and no cases have been reported in the U.S. Additionally, no increased incidence of neuropathy has been observed.

DRUG INTERACTIONS

Sulfonylureas

In a single-dose interaction study of type 2 diabetic patients, administration of metformin with glyburide did not result in changes in metformin pharmacokinetics or pharmacodynamics (9). Reductions in glyburide area under the curve (AUC) and C_{max} were observed but were extremely variable (9). Because this was a single-dose study and there is a lack of correlation between glyburide, serum concentrations, and pharmacokinetic effect, the clinical significance of this interaction is uncertain.

Furosemide

Metformin/furosemide interaction was studied in healthy subjects in a single-dose trial. This trial demonstrated that the pharmacokinetic parameters of both medications were affected by coadministration (9). Furosemide caused an increase in metformin's C_{max} and AUC (22% and 15%, respectively) without altering metformin's renal clearance. Furosemide's C_{max} and AUC were reduced by 31% and 12%, respectively. The terminal half-life of furosemide was reduced by 32%, without any significant alteration in renal clearance.

Nifedipine

Nifedipine apparently enhances the absorption of metformin. In a coadministration study with nifedipine, plasma metformin C_{max} and AUC were increased by 20% and 9%, respectively, while the time to maximum concentration (t_{max}) and the half-life were unchanged (9).

Cationic Drugs

An interaction between metformin and cimetidine has been observed in normal healthy subjects, with a 60% increase in peak metformin concentrations and a 40% increase in metformin AUC (9). However, in one single-dose study, the elimination half-life of metformin was unchanged. Metformin apparently has no effect on cimetidine kinetics. Other compounds that are eliminated via renal tubular secretion have the potential for causing an interaction with metformin by competing for renal tubular transport systems; therefore, these drugs should be used cautiously. Examples include amiloride, digoxin, morphine, procainamide, quinidine, quinine, ranitidine, triamterene, trimethoprim, and vancomycin.

Other

Metformin should be used cautiously with compounds that may lead to loss of glycemic control.

CLINICAL EFFECT

Monotherapy

In one 29-week randomized parallel double-blind trial of 289 moderately obese patients with type 2 diabetes, fasting plasma glucose levels were reduced by 58 mg/dl (3.2 mmol/l) on average, while HbA_{1c} levels were reduced by 1.8% on average in patients treated with metformin versus nutrition plus placebo (6). Fasting plasma glucose and HbA_{1c} in the metformin-treated group were 52 mg/dl (2.9 mmol/l) and 1.4% below baseline. Additionally, metformin was found to have an effect on plasma lipids in this trial, with triglyceride concentrations being reduced by 16%, LDL cholesterol by 8%, and total cholesterol by 5%. Also, there was an increase in HDL cholesterol of 2% (6). Patients treated with metformin in this trial lost a mean of 0.6 kg.

Another monotherapeutic trial of metformin evaluating dose-relationship response (500–2,500 mg) reported the greatest glycemic effect at a dose of 2,000 mg per day. In this trial, fasting plasma glucose levels were reduced by 86 mg/dl (4.8 mmol/l) and HbA_{1c} levels were reduced by 0.8% compared with baseline (13). Plasma lipid levels were not reported in this trial.

Metformin/Sulfonylureas

In a study of 632 patients with type 2 diabetes, metformin monotherapy was compared with glyburide monotherapy and metformin/glyburide combination therapy. These patients had previously been treated with sulfonylureas. In this trial, 213 patients were treated with metformin/glyburide combination therapy. The combination therapy patients had lower mean fasting plasma glucose levels (187 vs. 261 mg/dl [10.4 vs. 14.5 mmol/l]) and lower HbA_{1c} values (7.1 vs. 8.7%) than the patients treated with monotherapy. The effects of metformin monotherapy and glyburide monotherapy in this trial were similar (6). In this study, patients treated with metformin had statistically significantly lower levels of LDL cholesterol and triglycerides.

A trial of 55 patients with type 2 diabetes previously managed with insulin therapy assessed the feasibility of reimplementing oral therapy. Patients were treated with metformin and sulfonylureas. They all had a history of diabetes <30 years and had received insulin therapy for <10 years. Reinitiation of oral therapy was successful in 42 of the 55 patients and unsuccessful in 13. HbA_{1c} levels after successful reinitiation of oral therapy were significantly lower than baseline levels (a reduction of 1.3%). The patients in whom reinitiation therapy succeeded were those with shorter durations of insulin therapy, lower insulin requirements, and lower body mass indexes. The study concluded that successful conversion to oral antidiabetic therapy significantly reduced HbA_{1c} levels (14).

Repaglinide/Metformin

In patients treated with metformin in whom repaglinide therapy was added, a 40 mg/dl (2.2 mmol/l) reduction in fasting plasma glucose was reported compared with baseline treatment. Additionally, a 1.4% reduction in HbA_{1c} values compared with baseline was reported. Effects of this therapy on lipid levels and body weight were not reported (12).

Metformin/Insulin

Metformin/insulin therapy was studied in 50 insulin-treated obese type 2 diabetic patients who had previously failed to respond to sulfonylureas. During a 4-week run-in period, all patients were treated with placebo; they were then randomly assigned to continue placebo or receive active therapy with metformin (15). At 6 months it was reported that the patients treated with metformin/insulin combination therapy had fasting plasma glucose levels that were 91.5 mg/dl (5 mmol/l) below their blood glucose levels at baseline. Additionally, HbA_{1c} levels were reduced 1.9% below baseline treatment with insulin. Insulin doses in this trial were reduced by 25%, and the investigators reported reductions in total cholesterol and triglycerides and increases in HDL cholesterol.

Metformin/Acarbose

A study evaluating the effects of the addition of acarbose therapy in patients previously treated with metformin reported a reduction in fasting plasma glucose levels of 23 mg/dl (1.3 mmol/l) below levels in the metformin monotherapy group and a reduction in postprandial glucose levels of 62 mg/dl (3.4 mmol/l) compared with the metformin monotherapy group. Additionally, reductions in HbA_{1c} levels of 0.8% when compared with the monotherapy group were reported (16).

Pioglitazone/Metformin

Three hundred twenty-eight patients treated with metformin alone or with metformin and another antidiabetic agent were randomized to either pioglitazone (30 mg/day) or placebo. Metformin was continued, and other antidiabetic agents were discontinued. The addition of pioglitazone to metformin resulted in a mean reduction in HbA_{1c} levels of 0.8% and a 38 mg/dl (2.1 mmol/l) reduction in fasting blood glucose levels when compared with placebo (10).

Rosiglitazone/Metformin

Six hundred seventy patients treated with metformin were evaluated in two prospective randomized placebo-controlled combination metformin/rosiglitazone studies. In the first trial, metformin (2,500 mg/day) was continued and patients were randomized to receive placebo or rosiglitazone (4 or 8 mg/day). Fasting plasma glucose levels were reduced by 40 and 53 mg/dl (2.2 and 2.9 mmol/l) in the 4 and 8 mg/day groups, respectively, compared with placebo. HbA_{1c} was reduced by 1 and 1.2% in the 4 and 8 mg groups, respectively, compared with placebo (11). In the second trial, patients were randomized to combination metformin (2.5 mg/day) and rosiglitazone (4 mg bid) or were discontinued from metformin and started on rosiglitazone monotherapy. Fasting plasma glucose levels were reduced by 56 mg/dl (3.1 mmol/l) and HbA_{1c} was reduced by 0.8% in the rosiglitazone/metformin group compared with baseline.

REFERENCES

1. Bailey CJ: Biguanides and NIDDM. *Diabetes Care* 15:755–772, 1992

2. White JR: The pharmacological reduction of blood glucose in patients with type 2 diabetes mellitus. *Clin Diabetes* 16:58–67, 1998

3. Dagogo-Jack S, Santiago JV: Pathophysiology of type 2 diabetes and modes of action of therapeutic interventions. *Arch Intern Med* 157:1802–1817, 1997

4. Bailey CJ, Path MRC, Turner RC: Metformin. *N Engl J Med* 334:574–578, 1996

5. Stumvall M, Nurjhan N, Perriello G, Dailey G, Gerich J: Metabolic effects of metformin in non-insulin dependent diabetes mellitus. *N Engl J Med* 333:550–554, 1995

6. DeFronzo RA, Goodman AM: The Multicenter Metformin Study Group: Efficacy of metformin in patients with NIDDM. *N Engl J Med* 333:541–549, 1995

7. Bailey CJ: Metformin, an update. *Gen Pharmacol* 24:1299–1309, 1993

8. Yu JG, Kruszynska YT, Mulford MI, Olefsky JM: A comparison of troglitazone and metformin on insulin requirements in euglycemic intensively insulin-treated type 2 diabetic patients. *Diabetes* 48:2414–2421, 1999

9. Glucophage (metformin) package insert, Bristol-Meyers Squibb, 1998

10. Actos (pioglitazone) package insert, Eli Lilly, 1999

11. Avandia (rosiglitazone) package insert, SmithKline Beecham, 1999

12. Prandin (repaglinide) package insert, Novo Nordisk, 1998

13. Garber AJ, Duncan TG, Goodman AM, Mills DJ, Rohlf JL: Efficacy of metformin in type II diabetes: results of a double-blind placebo-controlled, dose-response trial. *Am J Med* 102:491–497, 1997

14. Bell DSH, Mayo MS: Outcome of metformin-facilitated reinitiation of oral diabetic therapy in insulin-treated patients with non-insulin-dependent diabetes mellitus. *Endocr Pract* 3:73–76, 1997

15. Gugliano D, Quantraro A, Consoli G, Minei A, Ceriello A, DeRosa N, Onofrio ED: Metformin for obese, insulin-treated diabetic patients: improvements in glycaemic control and reduction of metabolic risk factors. *Eur J Clin Pharmacol* 44:107–112, 1993

16. Chiasson J-L, Josse RG, Hunt JA, Palmason C, Rodger NW, Ross SA, Ryen EA, Tan MH, Wolevert MS: The efficacy of acarbose in the treatment of patients with non-insulin-dependent diabetes mellitus. *Ann Intern Med* 121:928–935, 1994

8. Insulin Use in Type 2 Diabetes and in Gestational Diabetes

INTRODUCTION

Patients with type 2 diabetes have defects in both insulin secretion and insulin action (1,2). Both defects are dynamic and lead to the clinical phenomenon of glucose toxicity. With the deterioration of glycemic control, there is a concomitant deterioration in the insulin secretory response. Furthermore, the impairment in insulin action at target cells increases the overall insulin requirement. Chronic hyperglycemia aggravates both the impairment in insulin secretion and the impairment in insulin action. However, with correction of the hyperglycemia, some improvement in the meal-stimulated insulin response, as well as improvement in insulin action, occurs. In other words, achieving glycemic control helps to maintain glycemic control.

Most patients with type 2 diabetes initially can secrete enough insulin to be treated effectively with nutrition and exercise alone or in combination with oral antihyperglycemic agents (3). However, as the disease progresses, the decline in insulin secretion may necessitate the addition of exogenous insulin. Data from the UK Prospective Diabetes Study (UKPDS) clearly demonstrate the progressive decline of glycemic control in patients with type 2 diabetes (4). After 3 years of monotherapy with a sulfonylurea, metformin, or insulin as monotherapy, ~50% of patients could attain the glycemic target of an HbA_{1c} <7%, two to three times the proportion of patients who could reach this goal with nutrition therapy alone. By the end of the 9-year follow-up, however, only ~25% of patients could attain the glycemic target with monotherapy.

INDICATIONS FOR INSULIN THERAPY IN TYPE 2 DIABETES

Additional findings from the UKPDS have led to the recommendation that insulin should not be the first choice for monotherapy in patients with newly diagnosed type 2 diabetes because it is associated with more hypoglycemic reactions and more weight gain (5). In addition, most physicians and patients prefer to institute therapy with oral agents (2).

When insulin is used as therapy in a patient with newly diagnosed type 2 diabetes, it is usually because of a markedly elevated plasma glucose level or primary failure of oral antihyperglycemic therapy (3). Patients with established type 2 diabetes are often given insulin either on a temporary basis for stress-induced hyperglycemia (e.g., due to acute illness or injury) or after secondary failure of oral agents. Other indications for insulin therapy in type 2 diabetes include (2):

- Development of severe hyperglycemia with ketonemia and/or ketonuria
- Uncontrolled weight loss
- Surgery
- Pregnancy
- Renal or hepatic disease
- Allergy or other hypersensitivity to oral agents
- Latent autoimmune diabetes in adults (LADA)

POTENTIAL PROBLEMS OF INSULIN THERAPY IN PATIENTS WITH TYPE 2 DIABETES

As in patients with type 1 diabetes, the primary adverse effects associated with insulin treatment in type 2 diabetes are hypoglycemia and weight gain (3). Weight gain during insulin therapy can be substantial, and the amount of weight gained generally can be correlated with the total daily dose of insulin (3). There is some clinical evidence that patients on some insulin regimens, such as bedtime insulin or preprandial insulin lispro, have a tendency to gain less weight.

Patients with diabetes who are receiving intensive insulin therapy appear to have less difficulty with hypoglycemia than do patients with type 1 diabetes on similar regimens. In addition, the use of the rapid-acting insulin lispro is associated with a reduced frequency of hypoglycemic events. In elderly patients with type 2 diabetes, insulin regimens should be designed to minimize the potential for hypoglycemia.

STRATEGIES FOR ORAL AGENT/INSULIN COMBINATION THERAPY

The results of clinical trials of combination regimens with the various oral antihyperglycemic agents and insulin indicate that insulin therapy may be beneficial for patients who fail to respond to treatment with combinations of oral agents or who fail to respond to insulin monotherapy (3).

For patients who cannot maintain adequate glycemic control on a combination of two (or more) oral agents, many physicians choose to initiate combination oral agent/insulin therapy by the addition of a single bedtime insulin dose, as in the bedtime insulin, daytime sulfonylurea (BIDS) regimen (3). Examples of the efficacy of some oral agent/insulin combination regimens, as demonstrated in clinical studies, are shown in Table 8.1.

For patients with type 2 diabetes who fail to maintain glycemic control despite large doses of insulin as monotherapy, control may improve with the addition of an oral agent (3). Because each class of oral agents has varied effects on body weight, plasma insulin levels, serum lipids, and insulin resistance, the selection of an oral agent for combination therapy can be tailored to the individual patient's needs, likelihood for compliance, need for weight control, and cardiovascular risk factors. Glimepiride, pioglitazone, metformin, and acarbose are approved by the FDA (Food and Drug Administration) for combination therapy with insulin (12). The goals of combination therapy are to improve the daylong glycemic profile by maintaining an HbA_{1c} <7% and to reduce the dose of insulin, the number of daily insulin injections, or both.

CONSIDERATIONS IN ORAL AGENT/INSULIN COMBINATION THERAPY

With the addition of new oral antidiabetic agents, including new sulfonylureas, thiazolidinediones, α-glucosidase inhibitors, and repaglinide, to the existing sulfonylureas and metformin, therapeutic decision-making for type 2 diabetes has become increasingly complex (13). Oral agents are often given in combination for additive efficacy; as a result, these therapeutic options have reduced the number of patients with type 2 diabetes who require treatment with insulin. The major question is the role of insulin in the treatment algorithm for type 2 diabetes.

Combination oral agent/insulin therapy is used for several reasons (14). First, virtually all patients with type 2 diabetes have fasting plasma glucose levels >140 mg/dl (7.8 mmol/L), and incorporating into an

Table 8.1 Efficacy of Oral Agent/Insulin Combination Regimens in Patients with Type 2 Diabetes

Reference	Oral/Insulin Combination	Baseline Mean HbA$_{1c}$	Mean Change in HbA$_{1c}$ with Therapy	Comments
Shank et al. (6)	Bedtime NPH + placebo Glipizide alone Bedtime NPH + glipizide	8.5% 8.2% 8.9%	–0.7% +0.2% –1.8%	Secondary sulfonylurea failures
Landstedt-Hallin et al. (7)	Preprandial regular insulin + glyburide Bedtime NPH + glyburide	9.2%	–2.1% –1.7%	Secondary sulfonylurea failures
Riddle and Schneider (8)	Insulin + placebo Insulin + glimepiride	9.9% 9.7%	–2.2% –2.1%	Secondary sulfonylurea failures; glimepiride/insulin restored glycemic control more rapidly and reduced insulin requirement
Giugliano et al. (9)	Insulin + placebo Insulin + metformin	11.5% 11.7%	–0.2% –1.9%	Secondary sulfonylurea failures
Coniff et al. (10)	Insulin + placebo Insulin + acarbose	6.6% 6.4%	–0.2% –0.6%	Treatment-naïve patients; acarbose/insulin reduced daily insulin requirement
Raskin and Graveline (11)	Insulin + placebo Insulin + troglitazone 200 mg Insulin + troglitazone 600 mg	9.43% 9.51% 9.32%	–0.1% –0.8% –1.4%	Patients previously on insulin; both doses of troglitazone/insulin reduced daily insulin requirement

existing regimen any pharmacological agent that will improve this state is a reasonable approach. Second, combination therapy may reduce the intensity of some of the adverse effects of insulin. Third, in most patients, glycemic control can be attained using combination therapy with an oral agent and insulin with a lower dose of exogenous insulin. Finally, the use of an oral agent in combination with insulin may help patients who are not responding to oral therapy alone to make the transition to insulin monotherapy and adjust to the idea of insulin treatment and the mechanics of a simple insulin regimen.

RATIONALE FOR COMBINATION ORAL AGENT/INSULIN THERAPIES

Sulfonylureas and Insulin

Sulfonylureas have been used in combination with insulin since their introduction (14). These agents lower blood glucose directly by stimulating the release of insulin from pancreatic β-cells and indirectly by sensitizing β-cells to glucose and increasing insulin secretion. The BIDS regimen has been shown to be effective in a several clinical studies (2,3). The dose of intermediate-acting insulin at bedtime decreases nocturnal hepatic glucose production and controls fasting hyperglycemia, while preprandial doses of a sulfonylurea stimulate the insulin secretory response to meals (2). BIDS therapy seems to be most beneficial for patients who are obese, have had type 2 diabetes for <15 years, were diagnosed after age 35 years, have a fasting plasma glucose level <250 mg/dl (13.9 mmol/L), and have residual insulin secretory ability (2,3).

A recent multicenter trial of glimepiride in combination with a single injection of evening insulin confirmed that this approach is safe and more consistently effective than insulin alone for obese patients beginning insulin therapy (15). In addition, a meta-analysis of 43 studies of sulfonylurea/insulin combination therapy concluded that this combination may be a more appropriate and suitable option than insulin monotherapy for long-term glycemic control in patients with type 2 diabetes who experienced primary or secondary failure with sulfonylureas (16).

Hypoglycemia and weight gain are common side effects associated with sulfonylureas and with insulin when each is administered as monotherapy (3). Most clinical trials of sulfonylurea/insulin combination therapy have not reported the rates of hypoglycemia during those trials, but the incidences of hypoglycemic episodes during sulfonylurea monotherapy are quite variable. The recent meta-analysis cited above indicated that glycemic control was achieved during sulfonylurea/insulin combination therapy without a significant change in body weight (16).

Metformin and Insulin

The oral agent metformin reduces fasting glycemia by decreasing glucose production in the liver (2,14). As a result, metformin can work in the presence of insulin and may facilitate its effects. At least one clinical trial has shown that the insulin requirement is significantly lower, by ~25%, during combination metformin/insulin therapy than during insulin monotherapy (17). Other studies have shown that the addition of metformin to an insulin regimen reduces the daily dose of insulin, the number of daily injections, and the levels of total and LDL cholesterol and does not increase body weight (12). A recent study comparing combination regimens of bedtime intermediate-acting insulin with glyburide, metformin, or both found that after 1 year, body weight remained unchanged and that there were fewer symptomatic hypoglycemic episodes among patients treated with metformin/insulin combination therapy, despite a comparable degree of glycemic control in the other groups (18).

The only reported adverse effects of metformin are gastrointestinal in nature, including abdominal bloating, cramping, nausea, and diarrhea (14). These effects are usually self-limiting and may be mitigated by gradual dose titration and by taking the medication with food.

α-Glucosidase Inhibitors and Insulin

The mechanism of action of the α-glucosidase inhibitors is to competitively inhibit the hydrolysis of complex carbohydrates in the small intestine, thereby reducing the absorption of glucose (14). In patients with type 2 diabetes, this action reduces postprandial glucose peaks and demands for insulin production (3,14). In addition, treatment with α-glucosidase inhibitors is not associated with weight gain. However, the results of a study of one α-glucosidase inhibitor, acarbose, combined with nutrition alone or nutrition plus sulfonylureas, metformin, or insulin suggested that the addition of this agent to insulin therapy provided only a modest improvement in glycemic control, with no significant changes in HbA_{1c} or fasting plasma glucose concentrations (19).

Gastrointestinal disturbances are the most common adverse effects associated with α-glucosidase inhibitor therapy (14). During combination therapy with insulin, complaints of flatulence, diarrhea, and abdominal pain are likely to occur. The treatment of hypoglycemic episodes during combination therapy may also be problematic, because the reduction in absorption rates of sucrose and other carbohydrates affected by α-glucosidase inhibitors may result in prolonged hypoglycemia. Such hypoglycemic episodes should be treated with glucose, not sucrose or complex carbohydrates (20).

Thiazolidinediones and Insulin

The thiazolidinediones appear to lower blood glucose levels by enhancing insulin action without enhancing endogenous insulin secretion (14). Given the correlation between insulin resistance and the risk of macrovascular complications in type 2 diabetes, the improvement in insulin resistance attributed to treatment with the thiazolidinediones may have a positive effect on hypertension and other cardiac risk factors. In obese patients with type 2 diabetes already receiving insulin therapy, the addition of a glitazone to the insulin regimen significantly reduced HbA_{1c} and fasting serum glucose concentrations and decreased the daily insulin requirement by >50% (21).

In general, glitazones are well tolerated. However, reports of severe idiosyncratic hepatocellular injury resulted in the removal of troglitazone from the market. See chapter 5 for more information. The two newer thiazolidinediones, rosiglitazone and pioglitazone, offer additional options for combination therapy with insulin, and neither agent has demonstrated signs suggesting a possible risk of liver toxicity, although liver function must be monitored. Rosiglitazone has been shown to significantly improve and maintain glycemic control over time by reducing insulin resistance and increasing β-cell function (22). Similar results have been seen with pioglitazone (23). Pioglitazone has been approved for use in combination with insulin.

INSULIN MONOTHERAPY IN TYPE 2 DIABETES

Patients with type 2 diabetes are classified according to the severity of their disease: mild, moderate, severe, and very severe (1). The degree of severity is based on the patient's level of fasting glycemia and ability to restore postprandial glycemia to basal levels, as a measure of the degree of meal-stimulated insulin secretion. Insulin therapy is virtually never needed for patients with mild type 2 diabetes, i.e., those with fasting plasma glucose levels <140 mg/dl (7.8 mmol/l) (1).

Insulin therapy is sometimes used for patients with moderate type 2 diabetes, i.e., those with a fasting plasma glucose between 140 and 220 mg/dl (7.8 and 12.2 mmol/L) (1). Basal insulin therapy is often sufficient for these patients, particularly if their endogenous insulin secretion is adequate to control postprandial glucose excursions. The basal insulin approach supplements endogenous basal insulin secretion and provides sufficient insulin to overcome the existing insulin resistance.

Basal insulin therapy is often administered as intermediate-acting (NPH or lente) insulin at bedtime, with or without a small morning dose (Table 8.2) (1). The peak effect of bedtime intermediate-acting insulin usually occurs before breakfast and thus controls fasting glycemia. Alternatively, basal insulin therapy can be given as one or two daily injections of a long-acting insulin. One of the new long-acting insulins, insulin glargine, has prolonged activity compared with NPH insulin and can provide basal insulin needs without producing the peaks of insulin action observed with lente and ultralente formulations (24). Most patients require a dose of ~0.3–0.4 U/kg/day (1).

Other insulin regimens may be designed according to the patient's individual glycemic profile (3). Some of the options include:

- NPH twice daily, mixed regular and NPH (or premixed 70/30 insulin) once or twice daily
- A more intensive regimen of multiple daily injections, such as premeal regular or lispro insulin with bedtime NPH
- Continuous subcutaneous insulin pump therapy

Patients with fasting plasma glucose levels >220 mg/dl (12.2 mmol/L) are considered to have severe type 2 diabetes, and they require the presence of exogenous insulin 24 h a day (1). Most patients with severe type 2 diabetes need to supplement the bedtime intermediate- or long-acting insulin with an additional dose of intermediate-acting insulin during the day or the addition of a short-acting insulin to attain adequate glycemic control. The total daily dose of insulin is usually in the range of 0.5 to 1.2 U/kg. Large doses, sometimes exceeding 1.5 U/kg/day, may be required initially to overcome the existing insulin resistance. High-dose therapy may be needed only to achieve glycemic control, which can then be maintained with lower doses of insulin, basal insulin therapy, or oral hypoglycemic agents. Insulin maintenance therapy is often continued at doses of 0.3–1.0 U/kg/day.

The rapid-acting insulin lispro appears to be superior to regular human insulin in patients with advanced type 2 diabetes (25). Clinical studies have shown that insulin lispro is effective in improving metabolic abnormalities in patients with type 2 diabetes by lowering fasting plasma glucose and postprandial blood glucose levels and by reducing postprandial blood glucose excursions, with no apparent increase in hypoglycemic episodes. Furthermore, insulin lispro restored early plasma insulin rise, improved glucose tolerance, and induced inhibition of hepatic glucose production.

Table 8.2 Comparative Time Course of Action of Insulin Preparations

Insulin Preparation	Onset (h)	Time to Peak Action (h)	Effective Duration of Action (h)	Maximal Duration (h)
Rapid Acting Lispro (analog)	<0.25	0.5–1.5	3–4	4–6
Short Acting Regular (soluble)	0.5–1	2–3	3–6	6–8
Intermediate Acting NPH (isophane)	2–4	6–10	10–16	14–18
Lente (insulin zinc suspension)	3–4	6–12	12–18	16–20
Long Acting Ultralente (extended insulin zinc suspension)	6–10	10–16	18–20	20–24
Combinations 70/30 (70% NPH/30% regular)	0.5–1	Dual	10–16	14–18
50/50 (50% NPH/50% regular)	0.5–1	Dual	10–16	14–18

From Skyler (1).

The fourth category of patients with type 2 diabetes, severe, is characterized by the lack of endogenous insulin response to meals (1). Patients with severe type 2 diabetes are unable to produce enough insulin to restore postprandial glycemia to basal levels within 5 h of meal consumption and may have fasting plasma glucose levels >250–300 mg/dl (13.9–16.7 mmol/L). The insulin secretory defect in these patients is so severe that it is often difficult to make a differential diagnosis from type 1 diabetes, with the exception of presentation with ketoacidosis. The initial approach to patients with severe type 2 diabetes is often similar to that for type 1 diabetes.

INTENSIVE INSULIN THERAPY IN TYPE 2 DIABETES

Type 2 diabetes is no less serious or debilitating a disease than type 1 diabetes, and intensive diabetes management, including intensive insulin therapy to meet glycemic targets, should be considered in appropriate patients (26). There is substantial and convincing epidemiological data linking hyperglycemia with an increased risk of macrovascular disease, a major cause of morbidity and mortality in patients with type 2 diabetes. Furthermore, the results of several prospective, randomized clinical trials, including the University Group Diabetes Program (UGDP) (27) and the UKPDS (28), show that intensive insulin therapy is effective for achieving glycemic control without adversely affecting cardiovascular mortality.

Type 2 patients using an intensive insulin regimen are managed in a manner similar to type 1 patients. The manufacturers of insulin pumps report that the fastest growing segment of insulin pump users are type 2 diabetes patients. Not all patients with type 2 diabetes, however, are appropriate candidates for intensive insulin therapy (26). The patients most likely to benefit from intensive diabetes management are those who:

- demonstrate competence and involvement in diabetes self-care
- are willing to become actively involved in daily management
- have a desire to improve glycemic control
- have mastered self-management techniques
- are willing to accept the risks as well as the benefits of intensive management
- can be open and honest with the diabetes management team
- recognize their physical and emotional abilities and limitations

- are willing to use health care and personal support networks

Conversely, intensive diabetes management is not appropriate for patients with type 2 diabetes who have the following medical characteristics (26):

- symptomatic coronary artery disease
- cardiac arrhythmias
- concomitant diseases or conditions that limit intensive management, such as debilitating arthritis or severe visual impairment
- relatively short life expectancy

Improved glycemic control is the desired outcome of any treatment of type 2 diabetes, including intensive insulin therapy (26). However, the benefits of intensive glycemic control must be weighed carefully against the demands of intensive management, the risks of weight gain and hyperglycemia, and the financial constraints in the current health care climate.

INSULIN USE IN GESTATIONAL DIABETES

Gestational diabetes mellitus (GDM) develops in 2–5% of pregnant women in the U.S. (29). Women with GDM are at increased risk for the development of type 2 diabetes later in life, and their infants are at risk for macrosomia, a major complication that can adversely affect both maternal and fetal outcome (30). Nutrition and exercise are integral parts of GDM management, and insulin therapy is aimed at reducing maternal hyperglycemia, fetal hyperglycemia and hyperinsulinemia, and macrosomia. For women with postprandial hyperglycemia, insulin treatment is usually initiated with a 30-U dose of a mixture of intermediate- and short-acting insulin in a ratio of 2:1 before breakfast. Initial insulin treatment for women with fasting hyperglycemia is often a bedtime dose of intermediate-acting insulin (10 U or less). Because many women with GDM are obese and insulin resistant, the insulin dosage is calculated on the patient's weight (30).

REFERENCES

1. Skyler JS: Insulin treatment. In *Therapy for Diabetes Mellitus and Related Disorders*. 3rd ed. Lebovitz HE, Ed. Alexandria, VA, American Diabetes Association, 1998, pp. 186–203

2. Skyler JS: Insulin therapy in type 2 diabetes. In *Current Therapy of Diabetes Mellitus*. DeFronzo RA, Ed. St. Louis, MO, Mosby, 1998, pp. 108–116

3. Feinglos MN, Bethel, MA: Treatment of type 2 diabetes mellitus. *Med Clin North Am* 82:757–789, 1998

4. Turner RC, Cull CA, Frighi V, Holman RR, the UK Prospective Diabetes Study Group: Glycemic control with diet, sulfonylurea, metformin, or insulin in patients with type 2 diabetes mellitus: progressive requirements for multiple therapies (UKPDS 49). *JAMA* 281:2005–2012, 1999

5. UK Prospective Diabetes Study Group: United Kingdom Prospective Diabetes Study 24: a 6-year, randomized, controlled trial comparing sulfonylurea, insulin, and metformin therapy in patients with newly diagnosed type 2 diabetes that could not be controlled with diet therapy. *Ann Intern Med* 128:165–175, 1998

6. Shank ML, Del Prato S, DeFronzo RA: Bedtime insulin/daytime glipizide: effective therapy for sulfonylurea failures in NIDDM. *Diabetes* 44:165–172, 1995

7. Landstedt-Hallin L, Adamson U, Arner P, Bolinder J, Lins PE: Comparison of bedtime NPH or prandial regular insulin combined with glibenclamide in secondary sulfonylurea failure. *Diabetes Care* 18:1183–1186, 1995

8. Riddle MC, Schneider J: Beginning insulin treatment of obese patients with evening 70/30 insulin plus glimepiride versus insulin alone: Glimepiride Combination Group. *Diabetes Care* 21:1052–1057, 1998

9. Giugliano D, Quatraro A, Menei A: Metformin for obese, insulin-treated diabetic patients: improvement in glycaemic control and reduction in metabolic risk factors. *Eur J Clin Pharmacol* 44:107–112, 1993

10. Coniff RF, Shapiro JA, Seaton TB, Hoogwerf BJ, Hunt JA: A double-blind placebo-controlled trial evaluating the safety and efficacy of acarbose for the treatment of patients with insulin-requiring type II diabetes. *Diabetes Care* 18:928–932, 1995

11. Raskin P, Graveline JF: Efficacy of troglitazone in combination with insulin in NIDDM (Abstract). *Diabetes* 46 (Suppl. 1):44A, 1997

12. DeFronzo RA: Pharmacologic therapy for type 2 diabetes mellitus. *Ann Intern Med* 131:281–303, 1999

13. Jacober S: Insulin therapy and combination regimens for type 2 diabetes. *Pract Diabetology*, June 1998, pp. 17–24

14. White JR Jr: Combination oral agent/insulin therapy in patients with type II diabetes mellitus. *Clin Diabetes* 15:102–112, 1997

15. Riddle MC: Combined therapy with a sulfonylurea plus evening insulin: safe, reliable, and becoming routine. *Horm Metab Res* 28:430–433, 1996

16. Johnson JL, Wolf SL, Kabadi UM: Efficacy of insulin and sulfonylurea combination therapy in type II diabetes: a meta-analysis of the randomized placebo-controlled trials. *Arch Intern Med* 156:259–264, 1996

17. Giugliano D, Quatraro A, Consoli G, Minei A, Ceriello A, De Rosa N, D'Onofrio F: Metformin for obese, insulin-treated diabetic patients: improvement in glycaemic control and reduction of metabolic risk factors. *Eur J Clin Pharmacol* 44:107–112, 1993

18. Yki-Harvinen H, Ryysy L, Nikkila, Tulokas T, Vanamo R, Heikkila M: Comparison of bedtime insulin regimens in patients with type 2 diabetes mellitus. *Ann Intern Med* 130:389–396, 1999

19. Chiasson J-L, Josse RG, Hunt JA, Palmason C, Rodger NW, Ross SA, Ryan EA, Tan MH, Wolever TM: The efficacy of acarbose in the treatment of patients with non-insulin-dependent diabetes mellitus. *Ann Intern Med* 121:928–935, 1994

20. Lebovitz HE: α-glucosidase inhibitors in treatment of hyperglycemia. In *Therapy for Diabetes Mellitus and Related Disorders*. 3rd ed. Lebovitz HE, Ed. Alexandria, VA, American Diabetes Association, 1998, pp. 176–180

21. Buse JB, Gumbiner B, Mathias NP, Nelson DM, Faja BW, Whitcomb RW: Troglitazone use in insulin-treated type 2 diabetic patients: The Troglitazone Insulin Study Group. *Diabetes Care* 21:1455–1461, 1998

22. Matthews DR, Bakst A, Weston WM, Hemyari P: Rosiglitazone decreases insulin resistance and improves beta-cell function in patients with type 2 diabetes (Abstract). *Diabetologia* 42 (Suppl. 1):A228, 1999

23. Schneider R, Lessem J, Lekich R, Pioglitazone 001 Study Group: Pioglitazone is effective in the treatment of patients with type 2 diabetes (Abstract). *Diabetes* 48 (Suppl. 1):A109, 1999

24. Coates PA, Mukherjee S, Luzio S, Srodzinski KA, Kurzhals R, Roskamp R, Owens DR: Pharmacokinetics of a "long-acting" human insulin analogue (HOE901) in healthy subjects (Abstract). *Diabetes* 44 (Suppl. 1):130A, 1995

25. White JR Jr: The pharmacologic management of patients with type II diabetes mellitus in the era of new oral agents and insulin analogs. *Diabetes Spectrum* 9:227–234, 1996

26. Farkas-Hirsch R (Ed.): Patient selection and goals of therapy. In *Intensive Diabetes Management.* 2nd ed. Alexandria, VA, American Diabetes Association, 1998, pp. 61–72

27. University Group Diabetes Program: Study of the effects of hypoglycemic agents on vascular complications in patients with adult-onset diabetes. II. Mortality results. *Diabetes* 19 (Suppl. 2):785–830, 1970

28. UK Prospective Diabetes Study (UKPDS) Group: Intensive blood-glucose control with sulfonylureas or insulin compared with conventional treatment and risk of complications in patients with type 2 diabetes (UKPDS 33). *Lancet* 352:837–853, 1998

29. Coustan DR: Gestational diabetes mellitus. In *Therapy for Diabetes Mellitus and Related Disorders.* 3rd ed. Lebovitz HE, Ed. Alexandria, VA, American Diabetes Association, 1998, pp. 20–26

30. Jones MW, Stone LC: Management of the woman with gestational diabetes mellitus. *Perinat Neonat Nurs* 11:13–24, 1998

9. Treatment of Hypertension in Patients with Diabetes

Hypertension worsens the prognosis for a patient who has diabetes. Diabetes and hypertension are each independent risk factors for peripheral vascular disease, cardiovascular disease, cerebral vascular disease, and microvascular disease. It has been estimated that complications in patients with diabetes may be attributed to hypertension in 30–75% of cases (1). Additionally, hypertension is two times more common in patients with diabetes than in their nondiabetic counterparts. Treatment of hypertension in patients with diabetes is generally more complicated than the treatment of hypertension in nondiabetic individuals. The choice of medication should include consideration not only of the impact of that medication on blood pressure but also of potential deleterious metabolic effects.

GOALS OF TREATMENT

Reduction of blood pressure in hypertensive patients has been shown conclusively to correlate with a reduction in cardiovascular risk and to slow or even attenuate the development and progression of microvascular complications (2). Several national consensus panels, including the current Joint National Committee on Prevention, Detection, Evaluation and Treatment of High Blood Pressure (JNC VI) and the American Diabetes Association, have recommended a goal of <130/85 mmHg for blood pressure reduction (1,3).

A number of clinical trials have demonstrated that blood pressure reduction is important and that special consideration should be given to the choice of antihypertension medication prescribed to the patient with diabetes. Unfortunately, aggressive hypertensive goals are not likely to be achieved by monotherapeutic interventions and many patients will require multiple medications in order to bring their blood pressure under control, as was demonstrated in the UK Prospective Diabetes Study (UKPDS) (4). In the UKPDS, hypertensive (>160/99 mmHg) patients were randomized to tight (<150/80 mmHg) or less strict hypertension control (<180/105 mmHg). The risk reduction afforded those with strict blood pressure control was significant, as is shown in Table 9.1. It was concluded that normalizing blood pressure is as important as normalizing blood glucose in reducing the complications of diabetes (4).

The treatment of isolated systolic hypertension in elderly patients with type 2 diabetes and in nondiabetic elderly patients was shown to reduce major cardiovascular events by 34%, stroke by 22%, myocardial infarction by 56%, and all-cause mortality by 26% in the SHEP (Systolic Hypertension in the Elderly Program) trial (5).

NONPHARMACOLOGICAL INTERVENTIONS

Several lifestyle modifications may be offered to patients with hypertension in an attempt to lower their blood pressure without drugs. These lifestyle modifications include (3):

1. nutrition therapy with the goal of weight loss if overweight
2. limited alcohol intake: no more than 1 oz (30 ml) of ethanol per day for men (e.g., 24 oz [720 ml] of beer, 10 oz [300 ml] of wine, 2 oz [60 ml] of 100-proof whiskey) and no more than 0.5 oz (15 ml) of ethanol per day for women and lighter-weight people
3. increased aerobic physical activity (30–45 min most days of the week)

Table 9.1 Results of Blood Pressure Lowering in the United Kingdom Prospective Diabetes Study (UKPDS)

Outcome	Risk reduction (P value)
Any diabetes-related endpoint	24% (0.0046)
Diabetes-related death	32% (0.019)
Myocardial Infarction	21% (0.13)
Stroke	44% (0.013)
Microvascular disease	37% (0.0092)
Two-step retinopathy	34% (0.004)
Reduction in visual acuity	47% (0.004)

4. reduced sodium intake: no more than 2.4 g sodium or 6 g sodium chloride per day
5. adequate intake of dietary potassium
6. adequate intake of dietary calcium and magnesium for general health
7. smoking cessation
8. reduced intake of dietary saturated fat and cholesterol for overall cardiovascular health

DRUG CATEGORIES

For a summary of the drugs available for the treatment of hypertension in diabetes, see Table 9.2.

Diuretics

Diuretics have been used widely for several decades as first-line agents in the management of hypertension. Of the diuretics, the most widely used are the thiazide diuretics. Thiazide diuretics have been shown to be very effective in lowering blood pressure when used in small doses (12.5–25.0 mg hydrochlorothiazide) (1). Additionally, these drugs have been shown to reduce cardiovascular mortality and morbidity in large, population-based, randomized, controlled trials. Thiazides are also effective in reducing the expanded plasma volume often associated with hypertension in diabetes.

Unfortunately, diuretics may cause several deleterious metabolic effects when used at higher doses. Glucose tolerance may be worsened with high-dose diuretic therapy (6). Deterioration in glucose tolerance in patients with diabetes usually occurs after 2–4 weeks of therapy, but it may occur after weeks or months of high-dose therapy in predisposed patients and may occur after months or years of therapy in patients without diabetes (6). The glycemic effects of diuretics depend on the type of diuretic, with thiazide diuretics having the most effect, followed by loop diuretics. Lastly, changes in glycemic control are not normally encountered with the use of potassium-sparing diuretics. The magnitude of diuretic-induced hyperglycemia is usually nominal; however, severe hyperglycemia and even hyperglycemic hyperosmolar nonketotic coma has occasionally been reported (6). Additionally, thiazide diuretics have been linked to mild elevations in LDL cholesterol and triglycerides, sexual dysfunction, and orthostatic hypotension, which may be particularly problematic in the patient with diabetes (7).

Table 9.2 Available Oral Antihypertensive Drugs

Drug	Trade Name	Usual Dose Range, Total mg/day* (Frequency per Day)	Selected Side Effects and Comments
Diuretics (partial list)			Short term: increases cholesterol and glucose levels; biochemical abnormalities; decreases potassium, sodium, and magnesium levels; increases uric acid and calcium levels; rarely, blood dyscrasias, photosensitivity, pancreatitis, and hyponatremia
Chlorthalidone (G)	Hygroton	12.5–50 (1)	—
Hydrochlorothiazide (G)	Hydrodiuril, Microzide Esidrix	12.5–50 (1)	—
Indapamide	Lozol	1.25–5 (1)	(Less or no hypercholesterolemia)
Metolazone	Mykrox	0.5–1.0 (1)	—
	Zaroxolyn	2.5–10 (1)	—
Loop diuretics			
Bumetanide (G)	Bumex	0.5–4 (2–3)	(Short duration of action, no hypercalcemia)
Ethacrynic Acid	Edecrin	25–100 (2–3)	(Only nonsulfonamide diuretic, ototoxicity)
Furosemide (G)	Lasix	40–240 (2–3)	(Short duration of action, no hypercalcemia)
Torsemide	Demadex	5–100 (1–2)	—
Potassium-sparing agents			
Amiloride hydrochloride (G)	Midamor	5–10 (1)	(Hyperkalemia)
Spironolactone (G)	Aldactone	25–100 (1)	(Gynecomastia)
Triamterene (G)	Dyrenium	25–100 (1)	—
Adrenergic inhibitors			
Peripheral agents			
Guanadrel sulfate	Hylorel	10–75 (2)	(Postural hypotension, diarrhea)

		Dosage range (frequency per day)	Comments
Guanethidine monosulfate	Ismelin	10–150 (1)	(Postural hypotension, diarrhea)
Reserpine (G)†	Serpasil	0.05–0.25 (1)	(Nasal congestion, sedation, depression, activation of peptic ulcer)
Central α-agonists			Sedation, dry mouth, bradycardia, withdrawal hypertension
Clonidine hydrochloride (G)	Catapres	0.2–1.2 (2–3)	(More withdrawal)
Guanabenz acetate (G)	Wytensin	8–32 (2)	
Guanfacine hydrochloride (G)	Tenex	1–3 (1)	(Less withdrawal)
Methyldopa (G)	Aldomet	500–3,000 (2)	(Less withdrawal)
Terazosin hydrochloride			(Hepatic and autoimmune disorders)
α-blockers			Postural hypotension
Doxazosin mesylate	Cardura	1–16 (1)	—
Prazosin hydrochloride (G)	Minipress	2–30 (2–3)	—
Terazosin hydrochloride	Hytrin	1–20 (1)	—
β-blockers			Bronchospasm, bradycardia, heart failure; may mask insulin-induced hypoglycemia; less serious: impaired peripheral circulation, insomnia, fatigue, decreased exercise tolerance, hypertriglyceridemia (except agents with intrinsic sympathomimetic activity)
Acebutolol‡ §	Sectral	200–800 (1)	—
Atenolol (G)‡	Tenormin	25–100 (1–2)	—
Betaxolol hydrochloride	Kerlone	5–20 (1)	—
Bisoprolol fumarates	Zebeta	2.5–10 (1)	—
Cateolol hydrochloride§	Cartrol	205–10 (1)	—
Metoprolol tartrate (G)‡	Lopressor	50–300 (2)	—
Metoprolol succinate‡	Toprol-XL	50–300 (1)	—
Nadolol (G)	Corgard	40–320 (1)	—
Penbutolol sulfate§	Levatol	10–20 (1)	—

(Continued)

Table 9.2 Available Oral Antihypertensive Drugs (*Continued*)

Drug	Trade Name	Usual Dose Range, Total mg/day* (Frequency per Day)	Selected Side Effects and Comments
Pindolol (G)§	Visken	10–60 (2)	—
Propranolef Hydrochloride (G)	Inderal	40–480 (2)	—
	Inderal LA	40–480 (1)	—
Timolol maleate (G)	Blocadren	20–60 (2)	Postural hypotension, bronchospasm
Combined α- and β-blockers			
Carvedilol	Coreg	12.5–50 (2)	—
Labetalol hydrochloride (G)	Normodyne, Trandate	200–1200 (2)	Headaches, fluid retention, tachycardia
Direct vasodilators			
Hydralazine hydrochloride (G)	Apresoline	50–300 (2)	(Lupus syndrome)
Minoxidil (G)	Loniten	5–100 (1)	(Hirsutism)
Calcium Antagonists			
Nondihydropyridines			Conduction defects, worsening of
Diltiazem hydrochloride	Cardizem SR		systolic dysfunction, gingival hyperplasia
	Cardizem CD, Dilacor XR, Tiazac		(Nausea, headache)
Mibefradil Dihydrochloride (T-channel calcium antagosist)	Posicor	50–100 (1)	(No worsening of systolic dysfunction; contraindicated with terfenadine [Seldane], astemizole [Hismanal], and cisapride [Propulsid])
Verapamil hydrochloride	Isoplin SR, Cafan SR	890–480 (2)	—
	Verelan, Covera HS	120–480 (1)	—
Dihydropyridines			
Amlodipine besylate	Norvasc	2.5–10 (1)	Edema of the ankle, flushing, headache, gingival hypertrophy

Drug	Brand	Dosage range (doses/day)	Side effects
Felodipine	Plendil	2.5–20 (1)	—
Isradipine	DynaCirc	5–20 (2)	—
	DynaCirc CR	5–20 (1)	—
Nicardipine hydrochloride	Cardene SR	60–90 (2)	—
Nifedipine	Procardia XL, Adalat CC	30–120 (1)	—
Nisoldipine	Sufar	20–60 (1)	(Postural hypotension, bronchiospasm)
ACE inhibitors			Common: cough; rare: angioedema, hyperkalemia, rash, loss of taste, leukopenia
Benazepril hydrochloride	Lotensin	5–40 (1–2)	
Captopril (G)	Capoten	25–150 (2–3)	—
Enalapril maleate	Vasotec	5–40 (1–2)	—
Fosinopril sodium	Monopril	10–40 (1–2)	—
Lisinopril	Prinivil, Zestril	5–40 (1)	—
Moexipril	Univasc	7.5–15 (2)	—
Quinapril hydrochloride	Accupril	5–80 (1–2)	—
Ramipril	Altace	1.25–20 (1–2)	—
Trandofapril	Mavik	1–4 (1)	—
Angiotensin II receptor blockers			Angioedema (very rare), hyperkalemia
Losartan potassium	Cozaar	25–100 (1–2)	—
Valsartan	Diovan	80–320 (1)	—
Irbesartan	Avapro	150–300 (1)	—

From the Joint National Committee on Prevention, Detection, Evaluation, and Treatment of High Blood Pressure (3). G, generic available.

*These dosages may vary from those listed in the *Physicians' Desk Reference*, 51st ed., which may be consulted for additional information. The listing of side effects is not all-inclusive, and side effects are for the class of drugs except where noted for individual drug (in parentheses): clinicians are urged to refer to the package insert for a more detailed listing.

†Also acts centrally.

‡Cardioselective.

§Has intrinsic sympathomimetic activity.

β-Adrenergic Antagonists

Although β-blockers have been shown to reduce cardiovascular morbidity and mortality in large, population-based, randomized trials, special consideration should be given to using a β-blocker in a patient with diabetes and to choosing a specific β-blocker. β-blockers have been shown to worsen glucose tolerance, and although this effect is typically mild, severe hyperglycemia has been reported in some cases (6). This effect is dose and duration related and is additive in patients with diuretic-induced hyperglycemia. Noncardioselective agents, such as propranol, have a greater effect on glucose tolerance than do cardioselective agents, such as atenolol. Drugs with intrinsic sympathomimetic activity, such as pindolol, have an even lesser effect on glucose tolerance. β-adrenergic antagonists have also been shown to have deleterious effects on lipid levels in some cases (1). Typically, triglycerides will be elevated while HDL levels will be reduced.

β-blockers have also been linked to an increased incidence of hypoglycemic episodes (6). More commonly, however, β-blockers, particularly noncardioselective agents, intensify hypoglycemia once it is present and delay its resolution. β-blockers blunt the counterregulatory effects of epinephrine, resulting in reduced glycogenolysis. These agents also cause an attenuation of hypoglycemic signs and symptoms, such as tachycardia, palpitations, hunger, tremor, irritability, and confusion. Perspiration, however, is usually enhanced and may serve as the hallmark of hypoglycemic episodes in patients treated with these drugs. Cardioselective agents such as atenolol tend to have lesser effects on hypoglycemic symptoms. β-blocking agents have also been linked to profound hypertensive states in hypoglycemic patients. This is due to unopposed alpha stimulation resulting from high concentrations of the counterregulatory hormone epinephrine (8,9).

Although the above-mentioned concerns should be considered when choosing an agent for the management of hypertension in a patient with diabetes, they must also be tempered by the recent findings of the UKPDS (4). In this trial, the cardioselective β-blocker atenolol was compared with the angiotensin-converting-enzyme (ACE) inhibitor captopril. The study reported that there were no differences in the blood pressure–lowering effects of these two drugs. Additionally, no statistically significant difference was observed in the incidence of cardiovascular endpoints, such as myocardial infarction, stroke, and congestive heart failure. The incidence of hypoglycemia was not statistically different between the two populations. However, additional glucose-lowering drugs were needed in 81% of patients treated with atenolol and in 71% of patients treated with captopril to control hyperglycemia after 8 years (10).

Although β-blockers are not contraindicated in the management of primary hypertension in patients with diabetes, the potential risks should be considered, and in most instances a cardioselective agent should probably be used if a β-blocker is deemed necessary (11). That being said, it should also be noted that β-blockers have been associated with reduced mortality in diabetic patients with known cardiovascular disease; therefore, for patients with known cardiovascular disease, β-blockers appear to be distinctly beneficial (12).

Calcium Channel Blockers

Calcium channel antagonists have been used in the U.S. for ~20 years. While these agents are widely used, their use is still under scrutiny. Short-acting dihydropyridines (e.g., nifedipine) have been associated with increased morbidity and mortality in some patient groups. Recently, the Appropriate Blood Pressure Control (ABC) study reported higher incidences of nonfatal and fatal myocardial infarctions in patients with type 2 diabetes who were hypertensive and taking nisoldipine, a long-acting dihydropyridine, than in similar patients treated with enalapril (13). There were no statistically significant differences between blood pressure levels in the two populations. This increased incidence in myocardial infarctions in the patients treated with nisoldipine resulted in discontinuation of that arm of the study by the Data Safety Monitoring Group. Unfortunately, this study was not empowered to test the effect of enalapril versus nisoldipine on cardiovascular outcomes. Therefore, the results of this study remain in question.

Two other studies, the Established Populations for Epidemiologic Studies of the Elder (EPESE) and the Multicenter Isradipine Diuretic Atherosclerosis Study (MIDAS), reported decreased survival and increased angina and cardiovascular events, respectively, in the patients treated with calcium channel blockers in those trials (13,14). It was suggested that the negative effects seen in these studies may have been due to the pharmacokinetics of short-acting calcium channel blockers. Recent studies, including the above mentioned ABC trial and the Fosinopril vs. Amlodipine Cardiovascular Events Randomized Trial (FACET), have both demonstrated a reduction in cardiovascular events in patients treated with ACE inhibitors versus patients treated with calcium channel blockers (15). While it should be remembered that these studies were not powered to evaluate directly the differences between these two drug categories on cardiovascular outcomes, the conclusions do warrant consideration.

Two studies evaluating dihydropyridine calcium channel blockers, the Syst-Eur trial and the Hypertension Optimal Treatment (HOT) trial, suggested no deleterious effects in patients with diabetes who were treated with calcium channel blockers (16,17).

Calcium channel blockers as a group have demonstrated no deleterious effects on either carbohydrate or lipid metabolism (10). In fact, verapamil has been reported to be associated with an improvement in glucose tolerance (18). One study reported a reduction in left ventricular hypertrophy along with a significant reduction in the risk of myocardial infarction in patients treated with ACE inhibitors and calcium channel antagonists (19). In fact, one author has suggested that the combination of ACE inhibitors plus dihydropyridine calcium blockers may provide the best outcome for patients with type 2 diabetes and hypertension; however, no prospective randomized trials comparing various combinations of antihypertension medications in patients with diabetes and their effects on cardiovascular risk have been carried out. Currently, a study is underway that will evaluate in a head-to-head fashion a dihydropyridine calcium channel blocker, a diuretic, a β-blocker, and an ACE inhibitor both in patients with diabetes and in patients without diabetes (20).

ACE Inhibitors

ACE inhibitors have assumed a prominent role in the treatment of hypertension and congestive heart failure since the initial development of the ACE inhibitor captopril in 1977 (21). Since that time, numerous trials have been carried out that have suggested the efficacy of these agents in the treatment of hypertension, congestive heart failure, and diabetic proteinuria.

One key study evaluating the effects of captopril in 409 patients with type 1 diabetes and proteinurea demonstrated conclusively that this medication was associated with a reduction in the risk of the combined endpoints of death, dialysis, and renal transplantation by 52% when compared with the rates of individuals with equivalent blood pressure reductions via other antihypertensive medications (22). Additionally, this study suggested that captopril offered renoprotective effects that were possibly independent of the effects of blood pressure reduction.

Another study in normotensive patients with diabetes reported a reduction in urinary albumin excretion and, more importantly, a postponement of the development of overt proteinuria over the 8-year study period (23). A total of 40% of the patients in the placebo group and 10% in the captopril group developed overt nephropathy.

A recent review of diabetic nephropathy in patients with type 2 diabetes concluded that ACE inhibitors were reasonable choices not only in the treatment of hypertension (as monotherapy and as combination therapy) but also in the management of proteinuria in these patients (24). These authors also concluded that calcium channel antagonists should not be administered as monotherapy. Based on currently available evidence, the use of ACE inhibitors in patients with type 1 or type 2 diabetes who have microalbuminuria, even in the absence of hypertension, is accepted (25). Additionally, ACE inhibitors have been promoted to be the drugs of choice for hypertensive patients with diabetes. A very relevant trial by the HOPE (Heart Outcomes Prevention Evaluation) Study investigators concluded that the ACE inhibitor, ramipril, significantly reduces the rates of death, myocardial infarction, and stroke in a broad range of high-risk patients who are not known to have a low ejection fraction or heart failure (26).

One concern with the use of ACE inhibitors in patients with diabetes has been the potential for the attenuation of their effectiveness with the concomitant use of aspirin. A recent study of over 11,000 patients concluded that the use of low-dose aspirin, i.e., <250 mg/day, in combination with ACE inhibitors is safe and in fact may be beneficial in patients who have coronary artery disease, regardless of their congestive heart failure status (27).

Angiotensin II Blockers

In general terms, angiotensin II blockers are well tolerated, cause no deleterious metabolic effects, and should be considered in patients with diabetic proteinuria who are intolerant to ACE inhibitors (3).

CONCLUSIONS

Although no single antihypertensive agent is best suited for all patients with diabetes, ACE inhibitors may offer an advantage over most of the other first-line agents for monotherapeutic treatment of hypertension because their use does not result in significant adverse effects on glucose or lipid profiles and because these agents appear to be renoprotective. It is important to consider not only the antihypertensive effect but also the potential deleterious metabolic abnormalities caused by any antihypertensive medication used. Lastly, the clinician should also consider that in many cases multiple antihypertensive medications will be required. Aggressive management of blood pressure, elevated blood lipids, and blood glucose should be an objective of treatment for all patients with diabetes.

REFERENCES

1. American Diabetes Association: Treatment of hypertension in diabetes (Consensus Statement). *Diabetes Care* 16:1394–1399, 1993

2. Marks JB: Treating hypertension in diabetes: data and perspectives. *Clinical Diabetes* 17:148–154, 1999

3. Joint National Committee on Prevention, Detection, Evaluation, and Treatment of High Blood Pressure: The Sixth Report of the Joint National Committee on Prevention, Detection, Evaluation, and Treatment of High Blood Pressure. *Arch Intern Med* 157:2413–2441, 1997

4. Turner R, Holman R, Stratton I, Cull C, Frighi V, Manley S, Matthews D, Neil A, McElroy H, Kohner E, Fox C, Hadden D, Wright D: Tight blood pressure control and risk of macrovascular and microvascular complications in type 2 diabetes: UKPDS 38. *BMJ* 317:703–713, 1998

5. Curb JD, Pressel SL, Cutler JA, Savage PJ, Applegate WB, Black H, Camel G, Davis BR, Frost PH, Gonzales N, Buthrie G, Oberman A, Rutan GH, Stamler J, the Systolic Hypertension in the Elderly Program Cooperative Research Group: Effect of diuretic-based antihypertensive treatment on cardiovascular disease risk in older diabetic patients with isolated systolic hypertension. *JAMA* 276:1886–1892, 1996

6. White JR, Hartman J, Campbell RK: Drug interactions in diabetic patients: the risk of losing glycemic control. *Drug Interactions* 93:131–142, 1993

7. Kimble MA: Diabetes mellitus. In *Applied Therapeutics: The Clinical Use of Drugs.* 4th ed. Young LY, Koda-Kimble MA, Eds. Vancouver, Applied Therapeutics, 1988, pp. 1663–1742

8. Shepherd AM, Lin MS, Keeton TK: Hypoglycemia-induced hypertension in a diabetic patient on metoprolol. *Ann Intern Med* 94:357–358, 1981

9. McMurtrey RJ: Propranolol, hypoglycemia and hypertensive crisis (Letter). *Ann Intern Med* 80:669–670, 1974

10. MacLeod MJ, McLay J: Drug treatment of hypertension complicating diabetes mellitus. *Drugs* 56:189–202, 1998

11. Pahor M, Guralnik JM, Corti M-C, Foley DJ, Carbonin P, Havlik RJ: Long-term survival and use of antihypertensive medications in older persons. *J Am Geriatr Soc* 43:1191–1197, 1995

12. Gottleib SS, McCarter RJ, Vogel RA: Effect of beta-blockade on mortality among high-risk and low-risk patients after myocardial infarction. *N Engl J Med* 339:489–497, 1998

13. Estacio RO, Jeffers BW, Hiatt WR, Biggerstaff SL, Gifford N, Schrier RW: The effect of nisoldipine as compared with enalapril

on cardiovascular outcomes in patients with non-insulin-dependent diabetes and hypertension. *N Engl J Med* 338:645–652, 1998

14. Borhani NO, Mercuri M, Borhani PA, Buckalew VM, Canossa-Terris M, Carr AA, Kappagoda T, Rocco MV, Schnaper HW, Sowers JR, Bond G: Final outcome results of the Multicenter Isradipine Diuretic Atherosclerosis Study (MIDAS): a randomized controlled trial. *JAMA* 276:785–791, 1996

15. Sowers J: Comorbidity of hypertension and diabetes: the Fosinopril versus Amlopidine Cardiovascular Events Trial (FACET). *Am J Cardiol* 82:15–19R, 1998

16. Tuomilehto J, Rastenyte D, Birkenhager WH, Thijs L, Antikainen R, Bulpitt CJ, Fletcher AE, Forette F, Goldhaber A, Palatini P, Sarti C, Fagard RH, the Systolic Hypertension in Europe (Syst-Eur) Trial Investigators: Effects of calcium-channel blockage in older patients with diabetes and systolic hypertension *N Engl J Med* 340:677–684, 1999

17. Hasson L, Zanchetti A, Carruthers SG, Dahlof B, Elmfeldt D, Julius S, Menard J, Rahn KH, Wedel H, Westerling S, the HOT study Group: Effects of intensive blood-pressure lowering and low-dose aspirin in patients with hypertension: principal results of the Hypertension Optimal Treatment (HOT) randomized trial. *Lancet* 351:1755–1762, 1998

18. Anderssen D, Rojdmark S: Improvement of glucose intolerance by verapamil in patients with non-insulin-dependent diabetes mellitus. *Acta Med Scand* 210:27–33, 1981

19. Messerli FH, Soria F: Ventricular dysrhythmias, left ventricular hypertrophy and sudden death. *Cardiovasc Drugs Ther* 8:S557–S563, 1994

20. Davis BR, Cutler JA, Gordon DJ, Furberg CD, Wright JTJ, Cushman WC, Grimm RH, LaRosa J, Whelton PK, Perry HM, Alderman MH, Ford CE, Oparil S, Francis C, Proschan M, Pressel S, Black HR, Hawkins CM: Rationale and design for the Antihypertensive and Lipid Lowering Treatment to Prevent Heart Attack Trial (ALLHAT). *Am J Hypertens* 9:342–360, 1996

21. White JR: From research to practice (Introduction). *Diabetes Spectrum* 6:170–200, 1993

22. Lewis EJ, Hunsicker LG, Bain RP, Rohde RD, the Collaborative Study Group: The effect of angiotensin converting enzyme inhibition on diabetic nephropathy. *N Engl J Med* 329:1456–1462, 1993

23. Mathiesen E, Hommel E, Smith U, Parving H-H: Efficacy of captopril in normotensive diabetic patients with microalbuminuria: 8 years follow up (Abstract). *Diabetologia* 38 (Suppl. 1):A46, 1995

24. Ritz E, Orth SR: Nephropathy in patients with type 2 diabetes mellitus. *N Engl J Med* 341:1127–1133, 1999

25. Cooper ME: Renal protection and angiotensin converting enzyme inhibition in microalbuminuric type I and type II diabetic patients. *J Hypertens* 14:S11–S14, 1996

26. Yusuf S, Sleight P, Pogue J, Bosch J, Davies R, Dagenais G, the Heart Outcomes Prevention Evaluation (HOPE) Study Investigators: Effects of an angiotensin-converting-enzyme inhibitor, ramipril, on death from cardiovascular events in high-risk patients. *N Engl J Med* 342: 145–153, 2000

27. Leor J, Reicher-Reiss H, Goldbourt U, Boyko V, Gottleib S, Battler A, Behar S: Aspirin and mortality in patients treated with angiotensin-converting enzyme inhibitors: a cohort study of 11,575 patients with coronary artery disease. *J Am Coll Cardiol* 33:1920–1925, 1999

10. Treatment of Hyperlipidemia in Patients with Diabetes

INTRODUCTION

Macrovascular complications are the most common cause of morbidity and mortality in people with diabetes in the western world (1). Fifty-five percent of deaths in people with diabetes are caused by cardiovascular disease (2). Patients with type 2 diabetes have a two- to fourfold increased risk of coronary heart disease (CHD) (3). Major risk factors such as hyperlipidemia, hypertension, and cigarette smoking markedly increase overall mortality caused by cardiovascular disease in people with diabetes (2). While it is clear that a multifactorial approach must be used in the prevention of macrovascular disease, management of hyperlipidemia is key.

A plethora of trials have demonstrated a strong link between hyperlipidemia and the development of macrovascular disease in patients with diabetes. The Multiple Risk Factor Intervention Trial (MRFIT), for example, investigated serum cholesterol levels as a risk factor for cardiovascular mortality in patients with diabetes. A subgroup of 5,163 men, aged 35–57 years at baseline examination, reported taking medication for diabetes. When compared with 342,815 men not taking medication for diabetes, the cardiovascular and CHD mortality rates were increased by approximately threefold in patients with diabetes after a 12-year follow-up period (4).

Compared with patients who do not have diabetes, both men and women with diabetes have a greatly increased risk of dying from coronary artery disease (5). The sex-linked protection against CHD possessed by premenopausal women is substantially lessened or even eliminated when these women have diabetes.

Lipid abnormalities occur in 11–44% of adults with diabetes (2), and atherosclerotic complications account for up to 80% of all mortality in people with diabetes (6). Proper prevention, screening, and treatment practices for hyperlipidemia may help reduce the substantial morbidity and overall mortality associated with atherosclerotic complications in this population.

Although there have been no specific trials comparing the effects of lipid-lowering therapy on diabetic morbidity and mortality, larger studies have been completed that include small subgroups of patients with diabetes. The Scandinavian Simvastatin Survival Study (4S) (7) showed a statistically significant reduction (55%; $P = 0.002$) in the incidence of major cardiovascular events in patients with diabetes treated with simvastatin. A 36% reduction in overall mortality from CHD was also evident. This reduction, however, failed to reach statistical significance because of the small number of patients with diabetes in the study.

Subgroup analysis of the Helsinki Heart Study (8) showed that diabetes patients treated with gemfibrozil had a 3.4% incidence of major cardiovascular events compared with a 10.5% incidence in diabetes patients treated with placebo. Again, the difference between the two groups was not statistically significant, possibly because of the small number of patients with diabetes participating in the study.

Recently, the High-Density-Lipoprotein Intervention Trial (HITS) suggested that the use of gemfibrozil in patients with low HDL levels but otherwise relatively normal lipid profiles is efficacious in the secondary prevention of CHD (9).

Although extrapolation of data from larger studies provides encouraging results, a specific trial involving patients with diabetes is clearly justified. Data gained from such a trial would undoubtedly raise awareness, emphasize preventive techniques, encourage proper screening, and provide practical guidelines for the effective management of hyperlipidemia in patients with diabetes.

ALTERED LIPID METABOLISM IN PATIENTS WITH DIABETES

The most common lipoprotein abnormalities found in type 2 diabetes include elevated triglyceride levels, increased VLDL levels, and reduced HDL concentrations (3,10). Total cholesterol and low-density lipoprotein (LDL) levels are normal or slightly elevated in most patients (10).

Individuals with type 1 diabetes and strict glycemic control show little overall difference in lipoprotein levels when compared with non-diabetic control subjects (11). Poorly controlled type 1 diabetes is associated with elevated triglyceride levels, increased VLDL levels, increased LDL concentrations, and decreased HDL levels (12,13).

The predominant causes of elevated triglycerides in both type 1 and type 2 diabetes include increased VLDL synthesis, impaired VLDL clearance, and reduced lipoprotein lipase (LPL) activity (10,12–14). The predominance of small, dense LDL particles in subjects with diabetes has also been identified. These LDL particles contain more triglycerides (10) and may be more atherogenic than the larger, less dense LDL cholesterol found in the nondiabetic population (15). Oxidation and glycosylation of LDL and other lipoproteins may increase their uptake into atherosclerotic lesions in diabetic patients (15). Elevations in the triglyceride content of HDL particles have also been observed (10). Obesity, smoking, and insulin resistance are contributing factors to lipoprotein alterations (1,13). Other identifiable factors thought to play a role in lipid abnormalities include nephropathy, renal insufficiency, and uremia (13,15).

DIETARY AND LIFESTYLE MODIFICATIONS

Lipid abnormalities associated with diabetes are often characteristic of inadequate control of blood glucose. Aggressive glycemic control should therefore be the primary goal in the treatment of diabetic dyslipidemia. Optimal diabetes control can be achieved through a combination of nutrition, exercise, weight loss, smoking cessation, and use of oral hypoglycemic agents and/or insulin if necessary.

Alterations in nutrition can improve insulin resistance in type 2 diabetes patients and in overweight type 1 diabetes patients (1). Controversy still exists regarding the appropriate percentage of calories that should be consumed as dietary protein, fat, and complex carbohydrates for people with diabetes. The American Diabetes Association (ADA) has established practical guidelines to help guide individual patients (13). In general, diabetes patients should reduce total caloric intake and saturated fat intake. Registered dietitians can provide valuable assistance to patients with diabetes, as well as to other health care providers, by supplying motivation and important information regarding food content and dietary exchanges.

Physical activity can bring about important metabolic changes in patients with diabetes. Changes in body weight and body composition lower triglyceride, total cholesterol, and LDL cholesterol levels while increasing HDL cholesterol levels. Exercise programs should be individualized in all patients with diabetes (11). Extensive motivation, support, and continuous follow-up are often required. Individualized programs should be tailored to the patient's diabetic complications, history, and medical status. Vascular complications may limit the amount or types of physical activity that can be implemented.

The combination of nutrition therapy and increased physical activity often enhances total weight loss and assists in overall weight maintenance. Weight loss is associated with improvements in triglycerides, insulin sensitivity, and glucose control; reductions in total and LDL cholesterol; and increases in HDL cholesterol (11). Generally, the greater the weight loss, the greater the improvement in these parameters, but even a weight loss of <10 lb has been shown to improve lipid patterns (11).

The role of smoking cessation and reduction of alcohol intake should not be ignored in this population. Smoking is a major risk factor for atherosclerosis, CHD, and myocardial infarction (16). Excessive alcohol intake can aggravate hypertriglyceridemia and thus negate any purported benefit to HDL cholesterol levels (15).

EFFECT OF GLUCOSE-LOWERING AGENTS ON LIPOPROTEINS

Insulin and oral hypoglycemic therapy, including metformin, thiazolidinediones, and sulfonylureas, are associated with improvements in glucose control, insulin sensitivity, and lipoprotein abnormalities. Metformin has documented lipid-lowering effects in patients with types 2 diabetes. Plasma triglyceride levels are decreased through reductions in VLDL cholesterol (1). Positive effects on LDL and HDL cholesterol have also been documented, but with less consistency (1). Oral sulfonylureas reduce total cholesterol and triglyceride concentrations in type 2 diabetes (1). Some studies show reductions in LDL cholesterol and improvements in LDL composition (1). Enhancement of lipoprotein enzyme activity and higher HDL concentrations have also been documented (1). Intensified insulin therapy can correct lipoprotein abnormalities in both type 1 and type 2 diabetes. Troglitazone, recently removed from the market, was linked to a modest decrease in triglycerides along with a slight increase in LDL and HDL (17). Pioglitazone therapy results in triglyceride reduction and an increase in HDL with no consistent changes in LDL or total cholesterol (18). Rosiglitazone therapy results in a reduction in free fatty acids and an increase in LDL and HDL (19).

GOALS FOR LIPOPROTEIN THERAPY

The categories of CHD risk based on lipoprotein concentrations in adult patients with type 2 diabetes are given in Table 10.1 (3). Lipoproteins should probably be measured annually in this population because of the dynamic effect of changing glycemic control on LDL, HDL, total cholesterol, and triglyceride concentrations.

The National Cholesterol Education Program (NCEP) Report of the Expert Panel on Blood Cholesterol in Children and Adolescents recommends that children with diabetes be screened after age 2 years (20). The

Table 10.1 Category of Risk in Adult Patients with Diabetes

Risk	LDL cholesterol	HDL cholesterol	Triglycerides
Higher	≥130	<35	≥400
Borderline	100–129	35–45	200–399
Lower	<100	>45	<200

From the American Diabetes Association (3).

ADA suggests that optimal LDL, HDL cholesterol, and triglyceride levels for patients with diabetes are <100 mg/dl, >45 mg/dl, and <200 mg/dl respectively. In female patients with diabetes, it may be preferable to have HDL cholesterol concentrations of even higher than 45 mg/dl, since women tend to have higher levels than men. Raising HDL levels with lipid-lowering agents in patients with diabetes can be difficult because the most effective agent is nicotinic acid, which can worsen insulin resistance in patients with diabetes. However, the thiazolidinediones have been shown to increase HDL concentrations predictably; for example, in one trial, pioglitazone (45 mg/day) resulted in an ~20% increase in HDL compared with baseline. Although thiazolidinediones are not recommended as lipid-altering agents, this ancillary effect may be important to consider when choosing antihyperglycemic agents in patients with lipid abnormalities.

The recommendations for treatment of elevated LDL cholesterol are given in Table 10.2 (3).

In most cases, pharmacological intervention should be implemented if behavioral changes do not result in sufficient LDL reductions. However, in cases where the patient has clinical CHD and a very high LDL level (i.e., (200 mg/dl [11.1 mmol/l]), the ADA recommends that pharmacological therapy be initiated simultaneously with behavioral interventions. The ADA recommendations for pharmacological treatment of patients without macrovascular disease with LDL concentrations of >130 mg/dl (7.2 mmol/l) are the same as current NCEP practices for patients with known vascular disease. This variation on NCEP guidelines is justified by the high incidence of CHD in patients with diabetes and by their inordinately high morality rate secondary to CHD (3).

In patients with hypertriglyceridemia, behavioral modification, with weight loss, increased physical activity, and moderation of alcohol consumption, should be implemented. In cases of severe hypertriglyceridemia (i.e., >1,000 mg/dl [55.6 mmol/l]), severe dietary fat restriction (<10% calories from fat) along with pharmacological intervention should be initiated to reduce the risk of pancreatitis. Improved glycemic

Table 10.2 Treatment Decisions Based on LDL Cholesterol Level in Adults with Diabetes

	Medical Nutrition Therapy		Drug Therapy	
	Initiation level	LDL goal	Initiation level	LDL goal
With CHD, PVD, or CVD	>100	≤100	>100	≤100
Without CHD, PVD, and CVD	>100	≤100	≥130*	<130

From the American Diabetes Association (3).
*For diabetic patients with multiple CHD risk factors (low HDL [<35 mg/dl], hypertension, smoking, family history of CVD, or microalbuminuria or proteinuria), some authorities recommend initiation of drug therapy when LDL levels are between 100 and 130 mg/dl. Caveats: *1*) Medical nutrition therapy should be attempted before starting pharmacological therapy. *2*) Since diabetic men and women are considered to have equal CHD risk, age and sex are not considered "risk factors." CHD, coronary heart disease; PVD, peripheral vascular disease; CVD, cardiovascular disease.

control is very effective at reducing triglyceride levels and should be optimized before the initiation of fibric acids. In cases where triglycerides are between 200 and 400 mg/dl, the decision to start therapy should be based on the clinician's judgment.

Table 10.3 suggests the order of priority for the treatment of diabetic dyslipidemia in adults (3).

PHARMACOLOGICAL MANAGEMENT

When dietary modifications, lifestyle changes, and strict glycemic control fail to adequately control diabetic dyslipidemias, pharmacological management with lipid-lowering agents is warranted. Medications commonly recommended for the general population to control hyperlipidemia may not be appropriate for patients with diabetes. Table 10.4 lists antihyperlipidemic agents currently available in the U.S. along with their relative cholesterol-lowering potential.

The following section evaluates potential benefits and drawbacks of the currently available agents for hyperlipidemia and provides usual doses and contraindications for the medications commonly used and accepted as antihyperlipidemics.

Table 10.3 Order of Priority for the Treatment of Diabetic Dyslipidemia in Adults

I.   Lowering LDL cholesterol
     First line: statins
     Second line: bile acid binding resins

II. Raising HDL cholesterol
     Behavioral interventions

III. Lowering triglycerides
     Glycemic control
     Fibric-acid derivative
     Statins are moderately effective at high doses in hypertriglyceridemic patients who also have elevated LDL cholesterol.

IV. Combined hyperlipidemia
     First line: improved glycemic control and high-dose statin
     Second line: improved glycemic control and high-dose statin and fibric-acid derivative*
     Third line: improved glycemic control and resin and gemfibrozil*; improved glycemic control and statin and nicotinic acid (glycemic control must be carefully monitored)*

From the American Diabetes Association (3).
*The combination of statins with nicotinic acid and especially with gemfibrozil may carry an increased risk of myositis.

ADJUNCTIVE AND SECONDARY THERAPIES

Estrogen

Women who take conjugated estrogens after menopause generally develop CHD later than those who do not take estrogen. Therefore, hormone replacement therapy has been used in the management of dyslipidemias in postmenopausal women with diabetes, particularly those with other indications for estrogen replacement therapy (e.g., prevention or treatment of osteoporosis). The cardioprotective effects are thought to be secondary to its beneficial effects on the lipid profile (22). Estrogen, with or without progestin, decreases LDL by 15%, increases HDL by 15%, and slightly increases triglycerides (22). Caution is warranted in patients with severe hypertriglyceridemia and in those in whom estrogen may exacerbate a medical condition, such as estrogen-receptor-positive breast cancer (22). Also, use of estrogen replacement therapy in women with an intact uterus should be accompanied by progestin therapy. Unfortunately, the efficacy and safety of estrogen therapy for lipid reduction has not been studied in postmenopausal females with

Table 10.4 Antihyperlipidemic Agents Currently Available in the U.S. and Their Relative Cholesterol-Lowering Potentials

Antihyperlipidemic Agent	Total Cholesterol	Triglycerides	VLDL	LDL	HDL
Niacin (Vit. B₃, Nicotinic Acid)*	↓	↓↓	↓	↓	↑↑
Colestyramine (Questran, Questran Light)	↓	→↑	→↑	↓	→↑
Colestipol (Colestid)	↓	→↑	→↑	↓	→↑
Gemfibrozil (Lopid)	↓	↓↓↓	→↑	→↑	↑↑
Clofibrate (Atromid-S)	↓	↓↓↓	↓	→↑	→↑
Lovastatin (Mevacor)	↓	↓	↓	↓↓	→↑
Pravastatin (Pravachol)	↓	↓	↓	↓↓	→↑
Simvastatin (Zocor)	↓	↓	↓	↓↓	→↑
Fluvastatin (Lescol)	↓	↓↓	↓	↓↓	→↑
Atorvastatin (Lipitor)	↓	↓↓	↓	↓↓↓	→↑
Cerivastatin (Baycol)	↓	↓	↓	↓↓↓	→↑

From Iltz and White (20).
* Denotes over-the-counter status
→↑ = No Effect or Modest Increase →↓ = No Effect or Modest Decrease
↑↑ = Moderate Increase ↓ = Modest Decrease ↓↓ = Moderate Decrease ↓↓↓ = Substantial Decrease

type 2 diabetes and dyslipidemia (23). Therefore, carefully conducted studies are needed before estrogen can be recommended for use as a lipid-lowering agent. However, in the patient who carries another indication for estrogen replacement therapy, its lipid lowering effect may be beneficial.

Levothyroxine

Hypothyroidism is a common secondary cause of hyperlipidemia. All patients with diabetes should receive periodic thyroid function screening in order to rule out hypothyroidism as an underlying cause of lipid abnormalities. Levothyroxine does not lower lipid levels in patients with normal thyroid function and should not be used as a treatment unless the patient is hypothyroid (22). Plasma triglyceride levels often decrease with levothyroxine therapy, probably because of increased VLDL clearance and improved lipoprotein lipase activity.

Antioxidants

A number of agents that possess antioxidant properties have been proposed as being beneficial in slowing the progression of atherosclerosis. Vitamins E and C and beta-carotene are antioxidants that may help prevent LDL oxidation and its subsequent uptake by macrophages (11). Two large-scale studies have demonstrated a correlation between significant risk reduction of cardiac disease and vitamin E consumption (24,25). Furthermore, numerous studies have demonstrated that vitamin E, when given in supplemental doses of 200–800 IU/day, carries virtually no toxicity (26). Given the low toxicity cost of vitamin E along with the high incidence and rapid progression of macrovascular disease in this population, many endocrinologists routinely recommend vitamin E supplementation to their adult patients with diabetes. Although this therapy should not take the place of antihyperlipidemic therapy when needed, it may be useful as adjunctive therapy.

Fish Oil

Fish oil (omega-3, or n-3, fatty acids) has received much media and lay press attention over the past few years. An observational study conducted in the Netherlands found that men who consumed at least 30 g of fish daily had a 50% reduction in cardiovascular mortality compared with those who did not eat fish (22). Another secondary prevention trial with 2,000 myocardial infarction survivors reported that all-cause mortality was substantially reduced in individuals who ate fish at least two or three times weekly (22). Fish oils may reduce serum triglycerides secondary to their rich content of n-3 polyunsaturated fatty acids (28).

Unfortunately, fish oil can cause substantial weight gain and can impair glucose tolerance by increasing hepatic glucose production and inhibiting insulin secretion (22). Fish oil should also be used cautiously in patients with bleeding tendencies or thrombocytopenia. One author has suggested that the combination of fish oil and a statin may be useful in some patients with high LDL and high triglycerides (28). However, in this setting, blood glucose must be carefully monitored to ensure continued glycemic control.

Niacin

Niacin, a water-soluble B vitamin, is recommended by the NCEP as first-line treatment for hyperlipidemia. Higher doses than the recommended daily allowance are needed to reduce cholesterol levels. Niacin lowers LDL by 10–25%, decreases triglycerides by 20–50%, and increases HDL by 15–35% (22).

Many patients with diabetes have hypertriglyceridemia and lower than average HDL cholesterol levels. Therefore, one could make an argument that niacin would be an ideal choice for the correction of diabetic dyslipidemia. This, however, is not the case. In addition to causing bothersome side effects (such as flushing, pruritus, dry skin, headaches, nausea, and epigastric pain), which can drastically reduce patient adherence, niacin possesses troublesome metabolic consequences that cannot be ignored. Clinically significant metabolic side effects in patients with diabetes include hyperglycemia (27), hyperuricemia (15), insulin resistance (12), and abnormalities in liver transaminase levels (15). Therefore, the use of niacin as first-line therapy in patients with diabetes is clearly not recommended. The ADA states that niacin should be reserved for patients with refractory dyslipidemias and used only after careful consideration, with extensive follow-up and metabolic evaluation.

Contraindications

Niacin is contraindicated in patients with significant or unexplained hepatic dysfunction, active peptic ulcer disease, or arterial bleeding. It is also contraindicated in patients with known hypersensitivity to niacin (28).

Dose

The usual adult dose of niacin when used for management of hyperlipidemia is 1–2 g, two or three times daily. Therapy can be initiated with 250 mg given after the evening meal. The frequency and total daily dose can be increased every 4–7 days until sufficient alterations in LDL and/or triglycerides have been observed or until a dose of 1.5–2 g/day has been reached. If lipids are not adequately controlled after 2 months at this dose, the dose can be increased at 2- to 4-week intervals until 3 g/day has been reached. Rarely, higher doses may be needed; however, doses generally should not exceed 6 g/day (28).

Bile Acid Sequestrants

Bile acid sequestrants, such as cholestyramine and colestipol, are ion-exchange resins that bind bile acids in the gastrointestinal tract, forming an insoluble complex that is excreted in the feces. Because cholesterol is the major precursor to bile acids, the liver compensates for this reduction by extracting cholesterol from the blood to synthesize replacement bile acids via an oxidative process (21).

Resin therapy reduces total and LDL cholesterol and has little or no effect on HDL cholesterol. The major disadvantage of bile acid sequestrants in patients with diabetes is that they often cause an increase in triglyceride levels. This deleterious effect on triglyceride concentrations makes this class of agents unsuitable for many people with diabetes, and because of this the ADA considers bile acid resins as second-line agents (3).

Some patients who are refractory to other medications or those patients with severe nephropathy may benefit from the use of bile acid sequestrants. Because bile acids are not absorbed systemically, they are some of the safest lipid-lowering agents for patients with diabetic nephropathy (12).

Bile acid sequestrants and niacin are the only antihyperlipidemic medications indicated for use in children and adolescents ≥10 years of age by the NCEP (12). It is reasonable to recommend resins as first-line therapy for individuals with type 1 diabetes who are 10–18 years of age. The growth and development of young type 1 diabetes patients should be closely monitored, and multivitamin supplements should be given because of the possibility of systemic deficiencies in fat-soluble vitamins and folate induced by high-dose resin therapy (12).

A frequent side effect of resin therapy is constipation. Therefore, this therapy should not be used in patients with autonomic neuropathy and severe constipation (12). Other more frequently noted adverse events that may lessen with continued therapy include flatulence, nausea, dyspepsia, and inability to tolerate the taste of the resins.

Patient education is of utmost importance when resin therapy is implemented. Bile acid sequestrants are known to interfere with the systemic absorption of many medications. Patients should be instructed to take other medications at least 1 h before or 4–6 h after cholestyramine or colestipol. Appropriate administration techniques and maintenance of hydration is vital to prevent constipation and fecal impaction in all patients.

Contraindications

Colestipol HCL is contraindicated in patients with known hypersensitivity to any of its components (29). Cholestyramine is contraindicated in patients with known hypersensitivity to any of its components and in patients with complete biliary obstruction (30).

Dose

In adults, the usual dose of colestipol HCL is 5–30 g/day given once or in divided doses (29). The usual starting dose is 5 g given once or twice daily. The dose may be titrated up by 5 g/day at 1- to 2-month intervals. To avoid esophageal distress and accidental inhalation, colestipol HCL should always be taken mixed with fluid and should never be taken in its dry form.

The recommended starting dose for Questran powder or Questran Light is one packet, or one level scoopful, once or twice daily (9 g Questran powder contains 4 g anhydrous cholestyramine; 5 g Questran light contains 4 g anhydrous cholestyramine) (30). Increases should be made gradually at intervals of 4 weeks. The recommended maintenance dose is two to four packets, or scoops, daily in two divided doses (although it may be given in one to six doses per day). The maximum recommended dose is six packets, or scoopfuls, daily. This product should always be mixed with water or other fluids before ingestion. The suggested time of administration is mealtime; however, this may be altered to avoid interference with the absorption of other medications.

HMG-CoA Reductase Inhibitors (Statins)

Several HMG-CoA reductase inhibitors (or statins) are used for the treatment of hyperlipidemia. HMG-CoA reductase inhibitors are appropriately named because they decrease the production of cholesterol by blocking the rate-limiting enzyme HMG-CoA reductase, which is responsible for cholesterol production. These agents are highly effective and better tolerated than other cholesterol-lowing agents.

Pharmacological benefits include upregulation of LDL receptors, enhanced LDL clearance, and reduced hepatic production of VLDL cholesterol (22). Clinical findings include substantially lowered LDL cholesterol, decreased triglycerides, and increased HDL cholesterol levels.

The HMG-CoA reductase inhibitors are especially valuable for diabetes patients with elevated LDL cholesterol and are considered first-line agents by the ADA (3). Findings from a small study in patients with diabetes involving the use of lovastatin (20 mg bid) showed a reduction in LDL levels by 28% and a decrease in triglycerides by 31% when compared with placebo (15). The greatest benefit was conferred in patients with the lowest baseline triglyceride levels (15). Simvastatin has also been evaluated in type 1 diabetes patients with established nephropathy. On average, LDL cholesterol was reduced by 37% (1).

Diabetes patients with elevated LDL cholesterol and mild hypertriglyceridemia are ideal candidates for HMG-CoA reductase inhibitors. The most recently approved agents, atorvastatin and cerivastatin, appear to have the most powerful LDL-lowering potential, without increases in adverse events. Patients with autonomic neuropathy may benefit from statin therapy because the lithogenicity of bile is reduced, thus curtailing their predisposition to cholelithiasis (12). Altered glycemic control has not been reported in diabetic patients using HMG-CoA reductase inhibitors. The risk of myopathy, although very small in the normal population, may be of increased concern in patients with diabetic nephropathy or moderate to severe renal insufficiency or in those concomitantly taking cyclosporine, gemfibrozil, or niacin (12). Careful monitoring is recommended, with frequent serial measurements of creatinine phosphokinase (CPK) and liver function every 6–8 weeks (12). Patients should be educated and instructed to report any signs of myopathy, including muscle pain, weakness, and/or tenderness, promptly, especially if accompanied by fever or malaise.

Contraindications

Statins should not be used in any patient with hypersensitivity to any component of these medications. They should not be used in patients with acute elevations or unexplained persistent elevations in liver function tests. These medications should be avoided in women of childbearing age who are likely to conceive (21).

Dose

The starting dose and dose range for these medications are given in Table 10.5. Therapy should be titrated at 4-week intervals (21).

Fibric Acid Derivatives

Gemfibrozil, fenofibrate, and clofibrate are the fibric acid derivatives currently available in the U.S. Fibric acid derivatives alter lipid metabolism through several possible mechanisms. They may decrease the hepatic production of VLDL cholesterol, increase lipoprotein lipase activity, enhance LDL receptor activity, and stimulate production of apoprotein A-I (4,13). Apoprotein A-I is thought to help maintain the integrity of HDL particles (13).

Beneficial effects of fibric acid derivatives include reductions in triglycerides and VLDL cholesterol, with subsequent increases in HDL cholesterol (13,15). Favorable compositional changes in HDL and LDL cholesterol are also realized (1). Mixed results concerning LDL cholesterol levels have been observed. Some studies suggest that fibrate

Table 10.5 HMG-CoA Reductase Inhibitors (Statins)

Generic (Brand)	Dosage Range	Starting Dose	Protein Binding	Elimination	FDA Approval Date
Lovastatin (Mevacor)	20–80 mg/day	20 mg hs	95%	Hepatic	1989
Pravastatin (Pravachol)	10–40 mg/day	10–20 mg po hs	50%	Hepatic	Oct. 1991
Simvastatin (Zocor)	5–40 mg/day	5–10 mg po hs	95%	Hepatic/renal	Dec. 1991
Fluvastatin (Lescol)	20–40 mg/day	20 mg po hs	98%	Hepatic	Dec. 1993
Atorvastatin (Lipitor)	10–80 mg/day	10 mg po qd	98%	Hepatic	Dec. 1996
Cerivastatin (Baycol)	0.2–0.3 mg/day	0.3 mg q hs	99%	Hepatic/renal	July 1997

hs, at bedtime.

therapy modestly reduces LDL concentrations (1), while others have reported transient or insignificant elevations in LDL cholesterol levels (4,15). The effect on LDL cholesterol may be correlated with the patient's overall triglyceride level (11). In general, patients with severely high triglyceride levels are more likely to experience less than favorable effects on LDL cholesterol.

Gemfibrozil has been used in this population with much success. As previously mentioned, in the Helsinki Heart Study, gemfibrozil showed a positive benefit in a subgroup of patients with diabetes, conferring a reduction in major cardiovascular events (8). Enrolled diabetes patients with mixed hyperlipidemia, including high triglyceride, high LDL, and low HDL cholesterol levels, had an overall reduction in coronary events of nearly 70%.

The so-called HITS trial was a secondary prevention trial in men with LDL ≤140, triglycerides <300, and HDL ≤40 mg/dl who were randomized to placebo or gemfibrozil (9). Approximately 25% of the 2,531 patients in this trial had diabetes. Gemfibrozil therapy resulted in a significant reduction (22% relative-risk reduction) in major cardiovascular events. This study suggests that the use of gemfibrozil in patients with low HDL levels but otherwise relatively normal lipid profiles is beneficial in the secondary prevention of CHD.

Other studies have shown improved fasting glucose and glucose tolerance in type 2 diabetes patients treated with a fibrate versus placebo (1). No significant changes in glycated hemoglobin were observed by these investigators.

Gemfibrozil is highly beneficial for diabetes patients with the most common lipid disturbances of elevated triglycerides, increased VLDL, and decreased HDL cholesterol. Patients suffering from severe mixed hyperlipidemia with elevated LDL may benefit from the addition of an HMG-CoA reductase inhibitor. Second-generation HMG-CoA reductase inhibitors, such as pravastatin and simvastatin, are recommended over first-generation agents, such as lovastatin, because of their low incidence of myopathy in combination with fibrates (4). Patients taking such a combination must be monitored closely for CPK elevations or the development of myopathy. Patients should be educated and instructed to report any signs of myopathy, including muscle pain, weakness, and/or tenderness, promptly, especially if accompanied by fever or malaise. The most common adverse events associated with gemfibrozil therapy are gastrointestinal disturbances, including dyspepsia, abdominal pain, and diarrhea. Taking doses immediately before the morning and evening meals can minimize gastrointestinal intolerance.

Clofibrate is rarely used, because of significant and consistent increases in the incidence of cholelithiasis. Clofibrate should be reserved for refractory hyperlipidemic patients who are not responding to other treatment modalities and in whom possible benefits from therapy significantly outweigh its associated risks.

Fenofibrate is the most recent addition to the fibrate class. Unlike gemfibrozil, fenofibrate has not been studied in combination with HMG-CoA reductase inhibitors (23,31). However, in one small trial of patients with diabetes, fenofibrate therapy resulted in a 40–50% reduction in triglycerides, an 11% reduction in total cholesterol, a 13% reduction in LDL, and an 8–10% increase in HDL (13). The reduction in LDL may have been due to an inhibitory effect of the drug on HMG-CoA reductase (13).

Fibric acid derivatives require a minimum of 3 months and probably at least 6 months to fully realize the maximum cholesterol-lowering effects attributed to therapy (11). Fibrates in general increase the risk of cholelithiasis and may need to be avoided in patients with impaired gall bladder motility due to progressive autonomic neuropathy. They are predominantly renally eliminated and should therefore be used with extreme caution or avoided in patients with severe diabetic nephropathy and chronic renal insufficiency because of an increased risk of myopathy.

Contraindications

Hypersensitivity to any component of clofibrate, fenofibrate, or gemfibrozil is a contraindication to therapy with a fibric acid derivative (31–33). Clofibrate is contraindicated in pregnant women, in patients with significant renal or hepatic dysfunction, in patients with primary biliary cirrhosis, and in nursing women (32). Fenofibrate is contraindicated in nursing women, in patients with significant renal or hepatic dysfunction, in patients with primary biliary cirrhosis, and in those with preexisting gallbladder disease (31). Gemfibrozil is contraindicated in patients with significant renal or hepatic dysfunction and in patients with primary biliary cirrhosis (33).

Dose

Clofibrate is given at 2 g/day in divided doses initially and for maintenance (32). Fenofibrate is given at 67 mg/day initially and titrated at 4- to 8-week intervals to a maximum of 67 mg three times daily (31). Gemfibrozil is given at 1,200 mg/day in two divided doses before the morning and evening meals (33).

CONCLUSION

Hyperlipidemia causes extensive morbidity and increased overall mortality in people with diabetes. Aggressive intervention strategies can help normalize lipid levels and undoubtedly decrease atherosclerotic complications in the diabetic population. Emphasis should be placed on preventative techniques and proper screening practices for diabetic dyslipidemia.

Initial treatment strategies include aggressive glycemic control incorporated with strict dietary changes and appropriate lifestyle modifications. If first-line treatments fail to control hyperlipidemia adequately, pharmacological interventions with cholesterol-lowering drugs are certainly warranted.

Medications should be chosen based on individual lipid abnormalities, concurrent disease states, side effects, and progression of diabetic complications. A thorough prevention, screening, and treatment program can help diabetes patients achieve their lipid-level goals and substantially reduce lingering disabilities, while increasing overall quality of life.

REFERENCES

1. Dean JD, Durrington PN: Treatment of dyslipoproteinaemia in diabetes mellitus. *Diabetic Med* 13:297–312, 1996

2. American Diabetes Association: *Diabetes 1996: Vital Statistics.* Alexandria, VA, American Diabetes Association, 1996

3. American Diabetes Association: Management of dyslipidemia in adults with diabetes (Position Statement). *Diabetes Care* 23 (Suppl. 1):S57–S62, 2000

4. Stamler J, Vaccaro O, Neaton JD, Wentworth D: Diabetes, other risk factors, and 12-yr cardiovascular mortality for men screened in the Multiple Risk Factor Intervention Trial. *Diabetes Care* 16:434–444, 1993

5. Vinik AI, O'Brian JT, Georges LP, Leichter SB, Janin Y: Management of hyperlipidemia in diabetes. *Compr Ther* 21:602–609, 1995

6. Lewis GF: Diabetic dyslipidemia: a case for aggressive intervention in the absence of clinical trial and cost effectiveness data. *Can J Cardiol* 11 (Suppl. C):24C–28C, 1995

7. Scandinavian Simvastatin Survival Study Group: Randomised trial of cholesterol lowering in 4444 patients with coronary heart disease: the Scandinavian Simvastatin Survival Study (4S). *Lancet* 344:1383–1389, 1994

8. Frick MH, Elo O, Haapa K, Heinonen OP, Heinsalmi P, Helo P, Huttunen JK, Kaitaniemi P, Koskinen P, Manninen V, et al.: Helsinki Heart Study: primary prevention trial with gemfibrozil in middle-aged men with dyslipidemia: safety of treatment, changes in risk

factors, and incidence of coronary heart disease. *N Engl J Med* 317:1237–1245, 1987

9. Rubins HB, Robins SJ, Collins D, Fye CL, Anderson JW, Elam MB, Faas FH, Linares E, Schaefer EJ, Schectman G, Wilt TJ, Wittes J: Gemfibrozil for the secondary prevention of coronary heart disease in men with low levels of high-density lipoprotein cholesterol. *N Engl J Med* 341:410–418, 1999

10. Lakso M: Dyslipidemia, morbidity, and mortality in non-insulin-dependent diabetes mellitus. *J Diabetes Complications* 11:137–141, 1997

11. American Diabetes Association: Detection and management of lipid disorders in diabetes (Consensus Statement). *Diabetes Care* 16:828–834, 1993

12. Garg A: Management of dyslipidemia in IDDM patients. *Diabetes Care* 17:224–234, 1994

13. Oki JC: Dyslipidemias in patients with diabetes mellitus: classification and risks and benefits of therapy. *Pharmacotherapy* 15:317–337, 1995

14. Betteridge DJ: Lipids and atherogenesis in diabetes mellitus. *Atherosclerosis* 124 (Suppl. 1):S43–S47, 1996

15. Gates G: Dyslipidemias in diabetic patients: is standard cholesterol treatment appropriate? *Postgrad Med* 95:69–84, 1994

16. Haire-Joshu D, Glasgow RE, Tibbs TL: Smoking and diabetes (Technical Review). *Diabetes Care* 22:1887–1898, 1999

17. Rezulin (troglitazone) package insert, Parke-Davis, 1999

18. Actos (pioglitazone) package insert, Eli Lilly, 1999

19. Avandia (rosiglitazone) package insert, SmithKline Beecham, 1999

20. The National Cholesterol Education Program (NCEP) Report of the Expert Panel on Blood Cholesterol in Children and Adolescents. *Pediatrics* 89 (Suppl. 1):525–584, 1992

21. Iltz J, White J: Clinical management of hyperlipidemia in diabetic patients. *Diabetes Spectrum* 11:88–93, 1998

22. Clark AB, Holt JM: Identifying and managing patients with hyperlipidemia. *Am J Man Care* 3:1211–1219, 1997

23. Garg A, Grundy SM: Diabetic dyslipidemia and its therapy. *Diabetes Rev* 5:425–433, 1997

24. Rimm EB, Stampfer MJ, Ascherio A, Giovannucci E, Colditz GA, Willett WC: Vitamin E consumption and risk of coronary disease in men. *N Engl J Med* 328:1450–1456, 1993

25. Stampfer MJ, Hennekens CH, Manson JE, Colditz GA, Rosner B, Willett WC: Vitamin E consumption and risk of coronary disease in women. *N Engl J Med* 328:1444–1449, 1993

26. Bendich A, Machlin LJ: Safety of oral intake of vitamin E. *Am J Clin Nutr* 48:612–619, 1988

27. White JR Jr, Hartman J, Campbell RK: Drug interactions in diabetic patients: the risk of losing glycemic control. *Postgrad Med* 93:131–139, 1993

28. Mosby's GenRx: *Niacin*. St. Louis, Mosby, 1999 (monogr. no. p-1607-9)

29. Mosby's GenRx: *Colestipol HCl*. St. Louis, Mosby, 1999 (monogr. no. p-565-566)

30. Mosby's GenRx: *Cholestyramine*. St. Louis, Mosby, 1999 (monogr. no. p-475-476)

31. Mosby's GenRx: *Niacin: fenofibrate*. St. Louis, Mosby, 1999 (monogr. no. p-1607-9: 909)

32. Mosby's GenRx: *Niacin: clofibrate*. St. Louis, Mosby, 1999 (monogr. no. p-1607-9:533)

33. Mosby's GenRx: *Niacin: Gemfibrozil*. St. Louis, Mosby, 1999 (monogr. no. p-1607-9: 1029)

11. New Products in Development for Patients with Diabetes

A number of new drug products for the treatment of diabetes and its complications are under development. Information on these agents was obtained by a review of the medical literature, abstracts from recent endocrinology and diabetes meetings, a survey conducted by Pharmaceutical Research and Manufacturers of America, and press releases from numerous information services. The products farthest along in development are described in some detail, those in the earliest phase of development are summarized in Table 11.1.

PRODUCTS FARTHEST ALONG IN DEVELOPMENT

AERx Inhaled Insulin

AERx Inhaled Insulin (Aradigm) is in phase II development for the treatment of type 1 and type 2 diabetes. AERx is a hand-held inhalation device used with various insulin formulations for pulmonary delivery of the insulin. The device contains a microprocessor that produces a consistent dose, regardless of the patient's breathing ability (1,2).

Exendin-4

Exendin-4 (Amylin Pharmaceuticals) is in phase II development for the treatment of type 2 diabetes. Exendin-4 is a synthetic compound similar to a 39–amino acid peptide isolated from the oral secretions of the Gila monster lizard (*Heloderma suspectum*). Intravenous administration

Table 11.1 Agents under development for the treatment of diabetes and its complications

Generic Name	Trade Name	Manufacturer	Phase of Development	Comments
AERx Inhaled Insulin		Aradigm	Phase II	Types 1 and 2 diabetes. AERx is a hand-held inhalation device used with various insulin formulations. Device contains micro-processor that produces a consistent dose, regardless of patient's breathing ability
AJ-9677		Dainippon/Takeda	Phase I	
Encapsulated Human Islets	BetaRx-H	VivoRx Pharmaceuticals	Phase I	Type 1 diabetes
Encapsulated Porcine Islets	BetaRx-P	VivoRx Pharmaceuticals	Phase I	Type 1 diabetes
Encapsulated Proliferated Human Islets	BetaRx-Pr	VivoRx Pharmaceuticals	Phase I	Type 1 diabetes
Encapsulated Islets		Desmos, Inc/ TheraCyte	Phase I	Type 1 diabetes; islet cells are encapsulated before transplantation
Exendin-4		Amylin Pharmaceuticals	Phase II	Type 2 diabetes
Exendin-(9-39)		Alanex Corporation	Phase I	Treatment of diabetes
Fidarestat		GlaxoWellcome	Phase I	Treatment of diabetic neuropathy
GI262570			Phase I	Type 2 diabetes
Glucagon-like peptide 1 (GLP-1)		Saxon	Phase I	Stimulates secretion of insulin, inhibits glucagon secretion, decreases hepatic glu-cose production, inhibits gastric emptying, and promotes satiety and reduces food intake in type 2 diabetes
HMR 4902		Hoechst Marion Roussel	Phase II	

(Continued)

Table 11.1 Agents under development for the treatment of diabetes and its complications (*Continued*)

Generic Name	Trade Name	Manufacturer	Phase of Development	Comments
HR 1799		Hoechst Marion Roussel	Phase III	
Inhale Pulmonary Delivery System		Inhale Therapeutic Systems/Pfizer	Phase III	Inhaler delivers fine-powdered formulation of human regular insulin into the lungs
Inhale Pulmonary Delivery System		Hoechst Marion Roussel/Pfizer	Phase III	Inhaled human insulin for treatment of type 1 and 2 diabetes
Insulin, sublingual	Oralin	Generex Biotechnology Corp	Phase II/III	Buccal and sublingual mucosal absorption for the treatment of type 1 and 2 diabetes
Insulin aspart	NovoLog	NovoNordisk	Approvable letter	Rapidly absorbed and short-acting insulin for use in type 1 and 2 diabetes
Insulin glargine		Hoechst Marion Roussel	Pending approval	Long-acting, once-daily basal insulin for use in patients with type 1 or type 2 diabetes
Insulin lispro	Humalog Pen	Eli Lilly		Prefilled insulin pen delivery device
Insulin lispro	HumaPen	Eli Lilly		Refillable insulin pen delivery device
Insulin lispro 25%/ insulin lispro protamine 75% suspension	Humalog Mix 25 Pen	Eli Lilly		Mixture of insulin lispro and insulin lispro protamine in a pen delivery device
Insulin lispro 50%/ insulin lispro protamine 50% suspension	Humalog Mix 50 Pen	Eli Lilly		Mixture of insulin lispro and insulin lispro protamine in a pen delivery device
Insulinotropin		Scios	Phase I	Type 2 diabetes
Metformin/ Glyburide		Bristol-Myers Squibb	NDA filed	Combination product containing metformin and glyburide

Generic name	Brand name	Company	Phase	Indication
Nateglinide	Starlix	Novartis	Phase III	Treatment of type 2 diabetes. Nateglinide stimulates insulin release from the pancreas similar to repaglinide
Pimagedine (aminoguanidine)		Alteon	Phase II/III	Treatment of progressive kidney disease
Pramlintide	Symlin	Amylin Pharmaceuticals	Phase III	Type 1 and 2 diabetes
Prosaptide TX14		Myelos Neurosciences	Phase II	Treatment of diabetic neuropathy
Recombinant Human Insulin, Inhaled	Humulin	Eli Lilly	Phase II	Type 1 and 2 diabetes
Recombinant Human Insulin, Oral		AutoImmune	Phase II	Type 1 diabetes
R149524		Janssen Pharmaceutical	Phase II	Treatment of diabetic gastroparesis
RWJ 241947		R.W. Johnson Pharmaceutical Research Institute	Phase II	
SDZ DJN 608		Novartis Pharmaceuticals	Phase III	Type 2 diabetes
Voglibose		Takeda America	Phase II/III	Type 2 diabetes
Zenarestat		Warner-Lambert	Phase III	Treatment of diabetic neuropathy
Zopolrestat	Alond	Pfizer	PhaseII/Suspended	Preliminary reports indicate zopolrestat has no improvement in the nerve function of patients with diabetic peripheral neuropathy. Development of this compound has been suspended for the treatment of peripheral neuropathy. However, it is still in phase II development for the treatment of diabetic nephropathy and cardiomyopathy

Information for the table was obtained from references 1, 44–46, and 55–65.

of the synthetic exendin-4 produces a sustained, enhanced insulin response during periods of hyperglycemia (3).

Exendin-(9-39)

Exendin-(9-39) (Alanex Corporation) is a truncated amide of exendin-4. It works as a partial antagonist of the glucagon-like peptide I receptor (4). Exendin-(9-39) is in the early phases of development for the treatment of diabetes.

Inhaled Pulmonary Delivery System

Phase III studies of Inhale Therapeutic Systems' Inhaled Pulmonary Delivery System (Inhale Therapeutic Systems/Pfizer) are ongoing. The inhaler delivers a fine-powdered formulation of human regular insulin into the lungs. The particles are <5 μm in diameter and dissolve in the alveoli, releasing the insulin so it can be absorbed and transported by the pulmonary vasculature. The powder is contained in blister packs and is delivered using a inhalation device (5).

Insulin Aspart

Insulin aspart (NovoLog; Novo Nordisk) is awaiting approval for use in the treatment of patients with diabetes for the control of hyperglycemia. It has a more rapid onset and a shorter duration of action than human regular insulin and is intended for administration immediately before meals. It should be used in regimens including longer-acting insulin.

Insulin aspart is an insulin analog in which aspartic acid has been substituted for the amino acid proline at the B28 position. It has reduced hexameric binding following subcutaneous injection, resulting in more rapid absorption (6,7). Insulin aspart retains the potency, receptor binding characteristics, activity, and variability of metabolic effect of human insulin (6–11).

A 30/70 mixture of insulin aspart and its protamine-retarded form has a more rapid onset of action and greater activity within the first 4 h after administration than a 30/70 mixture of regular human insulin and NPH insulin (12).

Peak insulin levels are reached 40–45 min after insulin aspart administration, compared with 80–90 min after regular human insulin administration. Peak insulin levels are also higher after administration of insulin aspart. Insulin levels decline more rapidly as well (6,7,9,10,13,14). The pharmacokinetics and pharmacodynamics of insulin aspart appear similar to those of lispro insulin and more similar to those of endogenous insulin in healthy subjects than to those of subcutaneously administered regular human insulin (9,10,15).

The effects of therapy with insulin aspart on glycemic control have been evaluated in a double-blind crossover study enrolling 104 male subjects with type 1 diabetes, 90 of whom completed the trial. The inclusion criteria required the patient to be between 18 and 60 years of age, to have a body mass index (BMI) <29 kg/m^2, and to have an HbA$_{1c}$ <9%. In addition, patients had to be using unmodified human insulin before meals plus NPH at bedtime for at least 1 month before enrollment. After a 4-week run-in period consisting of therapy with regular human insulin before meals and NPH at bedtime, patients were administered either insulin aspart or regular human insulin before meals and NPH insulin at bedtime for 4 weeks. The 4-week treatment period was then repeated using the other insulin preparation. Premeal insulin doses were administered just before eating, and injections were made using a pen injector. Insulin doses were adjusted to maintain premeal and 0200 blood glucose levels within the range of 72.1–126.1 mg/dl (4–7 mmol/l) and postprandial blood glucose levels <180.2 mg/dl (<10 mmol/l) in the absence of hypoglycemic episodes. Insulin doses did not differ between treatments.

The 24-h plasma glucose control achieved with insulin aspart was better than that with regular insulin, as assessed by excursions of blood glucose outside the normal range of 72.1–126.1 mg/dl (4–7 mmol/l). In particular, insulin aspart reduced excursions of blood glucose >126.1 mg/dl (>7 mmol/l), without an effect on excursions <72.1 mg/dl (<4 mmol/l). Daytime glycemic control was better with insulin aspart, but nighttime control was poorer. Home blood glucose monitoring improved postprandial blood glucose control after lunch and dinner without deteriorating preprandial blood glucose control. After lunch, blood glucose values were 115.3 mg/dl (6.4 mmol/l) during insulin aspart therapy and 145.9 mg/dl (8.1 mmol/l) during regular insulin therapy ($P < .05$). After dinner, blood glucose values were 129.7 mg/dl (7.2 mmol/l) during insulin aspart therapy and 158.5 mg/dl (8.8 mmol/l) during regular insulin therapy ($P < 0.05$). No difference in blood glucose control, as assessed by serum fructosamine, was observed. Hypoglycemic episodes requiring third-party intervention occurred less frequently during therapy with insulin aspart (20 vs. 44 events, $P < 0.002$), although the overall incidence of all hypoglycemic episodes was similar during the two treatments (9). Hypoglycemia was the most commonly reported adverse effect in clinical trials with insulin aspart, occurring with a frequency similar to or less than that with regular human insulin (9,10).

Insulin Glargine

Insulin glargine (HOE 901) (Hoechst Marion Roussel) is a long-acting once-daily basal insulin for use in patients with type 1 or type 2 diabetes. The bioactivity of insulin glargine is 100% that of human insulin (11,16). When it is administered intravenously, insulin glargine produces a blood glucose response identical to that of intravenous administration of regular human insulin (16). Insulin glargine behaves like regular human insulin with respect to insulin receptor binding and activity and insulin-like growth factor I (IGF-I) receptor mediated signaling (17–19).

Insulin glargine was created by the addition of 2-arginine at the C-terminus of the B-chain and the substitution of glycine for asparagine in position A21 (16,20,21). The addition of arginine shifts the isoelectric point from 5.5 to 6.8 (21). Movement of the isoelectric point closer to neutral than that of human insulin, which has a pH of 5.4, results in insulin with a prolonged action (11,16). When the isoelectric point is moved by adding positively charged amino acids, it makes the insulin less soluble at the neutral pH of the injection site, resulting in precipitation of the insulin at the injection site (11,16).

The glycine substitution in the insulin results in a more dense crystal structure with a lower water content (21). Insulin glargine precipitates at pH 7.4 in the subcutaneous tissue, forming crystals. The denser crystals result in slower crystal dissolution, causing slower release of insulin dimers and monomers into the bloodstream (21). Insulin glargine has been formulated as a clear solution rather than as a suspension, so there is less need for mixing to ensure homogeneity of dose (21).

The onset of action is ~1 h following subcutaneous administration (22). Full activity is reached within 4–5 h and persists at a constant effect for 24 h (16,23). No significant insulin peak effect is observed after subcutaneous administration (21–24).

NPH insulin, insulin zinc suspension (crystalline, Ultratard), and insulin glargine have been compared in a glucose clamp study in 12 healthy subjects. Peak levels of exogenous serum insulin (calculated from insulin concentration corrected by C-peptide estimate of endogenous production) were 25 μU/ml at 4 h after NPH insulin administration and declined thereafter. Exogenous insulin levels rose progressively to 9 μU/ml at 14–22 h after Ultratard administration. Exogenous insulin levels rose to 10 μU/ml at 5 h, with a plateau observed at points beyond 4 h after insulin glargine administration (23). In comparison with NPH insulin in another study, absorption of insulin glargine was lower in the first 4 h, but was comparable over the 30-h study duration (24). In another study, the onset (1.11 h vs. 0.71 h) and duration of action (22.8 vs. 13.8 h) of insulin glargine was increased approximately two-thirds compared with that of NPH insulin, and intersubject variability was reduced (22).

Similar absorption patterns are observed after subcutaneous administration into the leg, arm, and abdomen. The mean disappearance time for 25% of the dose was 11.9–15.3 h (25,26). In a study comparing absorption of insulin glargine and NPH insulin after subcutaneous injection into the abdomen, absorption of 25% of the dose was observed in 15 h for insulin glargine, compared with 6.5 h for NPH insulin (26).

Insulin glargine has been compared with NPH insulin in a study enrolling 534 patients with type 1 diabetes controlled with a regimen of NPH plus regular insulin. In addition to premeal injections of regular human insulin, patients received insulin glargine once daily at bedtime, NPH once daily at bedtime, or NPH twice daily for 28 weeks. The patients' blood glucose levels were well controlled before enrollment (baseline HbA_{1c} 7.7%), and only small reductions in HbA_{1c} were observed during the course of the study (–0.16% with insulin glargine and –0.21% with NPH insulin). Fasting plasma glucose was reduced to a greater extent in the insulin glargine group (–30.1 vs. –5.95 mg/dl [–1.67 vs. –0.33 mmol/l], $P = 0.01$). Hypoglycemia occurred less frequently in the patients treated with insulin glargine (39.9% vs. 49.2%). The incidence of both severe hypoglycemia and nocturnal hypoglycemia was lower in the insulin glargine group (27,28). Patients in this study treated with insulin glargine reported greater treatment satisfaction, improved perception of frequency of hypoglycemia and hyperglycemia, and a trend toward greater psychological well-being than did patients treated with NPH insulin (28).

Two insulin glargine formulations have been evaluated in comparison with NPH insulin in a 4-week study enrolling 256 patients with type 1 diabetes previously treated with a basal-bolus regimen. In addition to premeal injections of regular human insulin, patients received insulin glargine (containing 30 or 80 µg/ml zinc) once daily at bedtime or NPH insulin once daily at bedtime or twice daily, according to their prestudy regimen. At study entry, the mean fasting plasma glucose was 218 mg/dl (12.1 mmol/l) and the mean HbA_{1c} was 7.9%. After 4 weeks of therapy, the fasting plasma glucose was 165.7 mg/dl (9.2 mmol/l) on insulin glargine compared with 203.6 mg/dl (11.3 mmol/l) on NPH insulin ($P = 0.0001$). Lower basal insulin doses were required in the insulin glargine group. Hypoglycemia was common in all of the treatment groups, occurring at least once in 97% of the patients. Overall, adverse effects and injection-site reactions were comparable (29).

A similar study performed in Europe compared the two insulin glargine formulations with NPH insulin in 333 patients with type 1 diabetes previously treated with a basal-bolus regimen. As in the other study, patients received premeal regular human insulin plus insulin glargine (containing 30 or 80 µg/ml zinc) once daily at bedtime or NPH insulin once daily at bedtime or twice daily, according to their prestudy regimen. After 4 weeks of therapy, the fasting plasma glucose was 182.1 mg/dl (10.11 mmol/l) in the insulin glargine group compared with 216.2 mg/dl (12 mmol/l) in the NPH group ($P = 0.0001$). Self-monitored fasting blood glucose was 128.4 mg/dl (7.13 mmol/l) in the insulin glargine group compared with 142.7 mg/dl (7.92 mmol/l) in the NPH group ($P = 0.002$). HbA_{1c} was reduced by 0.14% in the insulin glargine group. The overall frequency of hypoglycemia was comparable between the groups, but nocturnal hypoglycemia occurred less frequently in the insulin glargine group than in the NPH once daily group (36% vs. 55%, $P = 0.0037$). No difference between the two insulin glargine formulations was observed (30).

Insulin glargine and NPH insulin have also been compared in 14 patients with type 1 diabetes. Patients continued to receive regular human insulin before meals. Nine patients received insulin glargine once daily at bedtime; the other five patients received NPH insulin twice daily. At 1 week and 4 weeks, the fasting plasma glucose was lower in the insulin glargine group (105.2 vs. 174.4 mg/dl [5.84 vs. 9.68 mmol/l] at 1 week, $P < 0.001$, and 111.1 vs. 166.5 mg/dl [6.17 vs. 9.24 mmol/l] at 4 weeks, $P < 0.01$). The insulin dose was reduced to a greater extent in the insulin glargine group. At the end of the 4-week study, HbA_{1c} was reduced 0.4% in the insulin glargine group compared with 0.2% in the NPH insulin group ($P > 0.05$) (31).

Insulin glargine has been compared with NPH insulin in a study enrolling 518 patients with type 2 diabetes treated with insulin. Patients received insulin glargine once daily at bedtime, NPH insulin once daily at bedtime, or NPH insulin twice daily for up to 28 weeks. Premeal regular human insulin was permitted as part of the daily regimen. Compared with the basal insulin dose before study initiation, the dose of basal insulin decreased by 1 U in the insulin glargine group but increased by 7 U in the NPH insulin group. The dose of regular insulin was increased in both groups. HbA_{1c} was reduced to a similar extent in the insulin glargine and NPH groups (0.41 and 0.59%, respectively). Fasting plasma glucose was also reduced to a similar extent (–31 mg/dl [–1.72 mmol/l] with insulin glargine and –21 mg/dl [–1.17 mmol/l] with NPH insulin). Weight gain was greater in the NPH group (3.1 vs. 0.9 lb, $P < 0.01$). Nocturnal hypoglycemia occurred less frequency in the insulin glargine group (31.3 vs. 40.2%, $P < 0.02$) (32).

Two formulations of insulin glargine have been evaluated in comparison with NPH insulin in 157 patients with type 2 diabetes inadequately controlled on a maximal dose of a sulfonylurea or a sulfonylurea plus metformin. The oral agents were discontinued, and insulin glargine (30 or 80 µg/ml zinc) or NPH insulin was given once daily at bedtime and individually titrated. Therapy was continued for 4 weeks. Fasting plasma glucose was reduced by 46.8–50.4 mg/dl (2.6–2.8 mmol/l) in the insulin glargine groups and 41.4 mg/dl (2.3 mmol/l) in the NPH insulin group. All subjects showed a marked improvement in fasting plasma glucose. There was no difference between therapies in fasting plasma glucose, fructosamine, HbA_{1c}, or frequency of hypoglycemia (33).

The two formulations of insulin glargine have also been evaluated in comparison with NPH insulin as an adjunct to therapy in 204 patients with type 2 diabetes moderately controlled on oral agents. Enrolled patients had an HbA_{1c} greater than 7%, were 40–80 years of age, had a BMI of 21–35, and were currently taking a sulfonylurea either alone or in combination with metformin or acarbose. There was no difference in glycemic control between the treatment groups. The HbA_{1c} was reduced by 0.8% from baseline in all three groups ($P < 0.0001$). Hypoglycemia occurred in 7.3% of insulin glargine–treated patients compared with 19.1% of NPH-treated patients ($P < 0.037$) (34).

Overall adverse effects observed in clinical trials were similar to those of NPH insulin (16,30,32). In one study, insulin glargine caused more pain at the injection site than did NPH insulin (20,32). The overall incidence of hypoglycemia was similar to or slightly lower than that with NPH insulin, although insulin glargine may be associated with less nocturnal hypoglycemia than once-daily NPH insulin (27,28,30,32).

Nateglinide

Nateglinide (Starlix; Novartis) will be used in the treatment of type 2 diabetes. Nateglinide stimulates insulin release from the pancreas in a manner similar to repaglinide. It has a quick onset and short duration of action (35–40).

A single-dose comparison of nateglinide, placebo, and repaglinide was conducted in 14 healthy subjects. The results of this study indicated that nateglinide (120 mg) was more effective than placebo, 0.5 mg repaglinide, and 2 mg repaglinide in lowering mealtime glycemia. It also had a quicker onset of action and a shorter duration of effect on the β-cell of the pancreas than did repaglinide. The effects of nateglinide may be more similar to physiological control of mealtime glycemia and may expose the patient to less insulin and decrease the risk of hypoglycemia (41). A 7-day placebo-controlled, double-blind, randomized, escalating, multiple-dose study continued to demonstrate the short acting effects of nateglinide on prandial glycemia, the improvements in glucose parameters, and no cases of hypoglycemia (42).

A double-blind controlled study was conducted in 289 patients with type 2 diabetes. After a single-blind, 4-week run-in period, patients were randomly assigned to treatment with placebo or nateglinide (30, 60, 120, or 180 mg) for 12 weeks. The medication was taken 10 min before the main meals of the day, and plasma insulin and glucose were determined. Nateglinide produced a rapid dose-dependent increase in insulin secretion, which peaked at 30 min, and a decrease in prandial glycemia. The baseline HbA_{1c} ranged from 6.8 to 10.5%, and the fasting plasma glucose was >140.5 mg/dl (>7.8 mmol/l) before the study.

The HbA_{1c} decreased by 0.04% with the placebo ($n = 60$), 0.23% with 30 mg nateglinide ($n = 51$), 0.37% with 60 mg nateglinide ($n = 58$), 0.59% with 120 mg nateglinide ($n = 62$), and 0.59 with 180 mg nateglinide after 12 weeks of therapy. The fasting plasma glucose was unchanged after 12 weeks of placebo therapy, but it decreased by 9.37 mg/dl (0.52 mmol/l) with 30 mg nateglinide, by 8.65 mg/dl (0.48 mmol/l) with 60 mg nateglinide, 15.1 mg/dl (0.84 mmol/l) with 120 mg nateglinide, and 10.3 mg/dl (0.57 mmol/l) with 180 mg nateglinide (35). Adverse effects included increased sweating, tremor, dizziness, and appetite and asthenia.

Pimagedine

Pimagedine (aminoguanidine) (Alteon) is in phase II/III development for the treatment of progressive diabetic kidney disease. Pimagedine interferes with nonenzymatic glycosylation and reduces levels of advanced glycosylation end products (AGEs). By decreasing AGE levels, pimagedine might be useful in preventing and treating other diabetic complications such as dyslipidemia, neuropathy, and retinopathy (43).

Pimagedine is well absorbed after oral administration. The volume of distribution is 1 l/kg. The majority of the drug is eliminated unchanged in the urine. The elimination half-life is 4 h in patients with normal renal function. The half-life increases with decreasing renal function and has been reported to be 38 h in patients with chronic renal failure (44).

Headache is the most common side effect of pimagedine. Dizziness has also been reported (44).

Pramlintide

Pramlintide (Symlin; Amylin Pharmaceuticals) is in phase III development for the treatment of type 1 and 2 diabetes (45). It is a stable, nonaggregating analog of endogenous amylin, a peptide secreted from pancreatic β-cells with insulin. It appears to delay gastric emptying and may regulate glucagon release, resulting in decreased postprandial hyperglycemia (44,46,47).

Peak serum concentrations occur within 30 min after subcutaneous injection of pramlintide. The volume of distribution is 56 liters. The elimination half-life is 30–50 min (44).

The impact of subcutaneous administration of pramlintide on metabolic control in patients with type 2 diabetes using insulin was assessed in a 4-week study. Two hundred three patients were enrolled in this randomized double-blind placebo-controlled parallel-group multicenter trial. Patients were treated with 30 μg pramlintide four times daily, 60 μg pramlintide three times daily, or 60 μg pramlintide four times daily. Serum fructosamine concentrations were decreased by 17.5 µmol/l with 30 µg pramlintide four times daily, by 24.1 µmol/l with 60 µg pramlintide three times daily, and by 22.6 µmol/l with 60 µg pramlintide four times daily, whereas the placebo produced a 3.5 µmol/l decrease in the serum fructosamine concentration. The HbA_{1c} decreased by 0.53% in the group taking 30 µg pramlintide four times daily, 0.58% in the group taking 60 µg pramlintide three times daily, and 0.51% in the group taking 60 µg pramlintide four times daily. The placebo reduced the HbA_{1c} by 0.27%. The total cholesterol concentrations improved with all three doses of pramlintide and only slightly with the placebo therapy (47).

A multicenter, double-blind, placebo-controlled study was conducted to evaluate the effects of concomitant pramlintide and insulin therapy on metabolic control in people with type 1 diabetes. A total of 586 patients were treated with subcutaneous insulin and pramlintide or placebo. Patients were randomized to treatment with 60 µg pramlintide three times daily, 90 µg pramlintide twice daily, 90 µg pramlintide three times daily, or placebo three times daily for 26 weeks. The mean baseline HbA_{1c} was 9%. The change in HbA_{1c} after 26 weeks was 0.1% with placebo, –0.2% with 60 µg pramlintide three times daily, –0.1% with 90 µg pramlintide twice daily, and 0.1% with 90 µg pramlintide three times daily. The mean change in body weight was 0.3, 1.6, –0.7, and 1.6 kg, respectively (48).

A 2-year multicenter study was conducted to evaluate the long-term effects of pramlintide plus insulin on glycemic control in people with type 1 diabetes. During the first year, the patients ($n = 480$) were treated in a double-blind, placebo-controlled study with placebo or 30 µg pramlintide four times daily. During the second year, the patients were treated with 30 µg pramlintide four times daily in an open-label extension study. The baseline HbA_{1c} was 8.8% in the double-blind portion of the study, and the mean change in HbA_{1c} at the end of the first year was –0.40% with pramlintide and –0.15% with placebo ($P = 0.0118$). One hundred twenty-six patients previously treated with pramlintide enrolled in the open-label phase of the study. The reduction in the HbA_{1c} during the first year (0.43%) was maintained throughout the second year of the study (0.35%) (49).

Adverse effects of pramlintide have included headache, lightheadedness, nausea, diarrhea, vomiting, and anorexia (44,48,49).

Prosaptide TX14

Prosaptide TX14 (Myelos Neurosciences) is in phase II development for the treatment of diabetic neuropathy (1). Prosaptide TX14 may prevent cell death and increase extracellular-regulated kinase phosphorylation and sulfatide content in primary Schwann cells or oligodendrocytes.

In addition, prosaptide TX14 may help in preventing degeneration and promoting regeneration of peripheral nerves (50).

Voglibose

Voglibose (Takeda America) is an α-glucosidase inhibitor that is in phase II/III development for the treatment of type 2 diabetes. Its mechanism of action is similar to that of acarbose and miglitol. By delaying the absorption of glucose from food, voglibose is able to improve postprandial hyperglycemia and fasting blood glucose (44).

An open prospective study was conducted in 27 patients with type 2 diabetes to evaluate the effectiveness of voglibose. Patients were divided into two groups; 14 were assigned to treatment with voglibose, and 13 served as a control group. In addition to the voglibose, the patients were treated with nutrition therapy alone or a sulfonylurea drug. Metabolic parameters were evaluated before treatment and at week 4 of treatment. At the end of the fourth week, HbA_{1c} and plasma glucose were similar in both groups. However, insulin secretion, as measured by area under the curve of daily serum insulin, was improved (51).

A randomized, placebo-controlled, double-masked, fivefold crossover study was conducted with 20 healthy male volunteers. This study was conducted to compare the impact of acarbose and voglibose on plasma immunoreactive insulin, plasma glucose, and 24-h urinary connecting peptide immunoreactivity excretion. Both acarbose and voglibose decreased the postprandial increase in plasma glucose level, but the reduction was small. The maximum concentration and area under the plasma concentration-time curve of plasma immunoreactive insulin after meals decreased with both drugs. Urinary connecting peptide immunoreactivity excretion was decreased by 30.6% with 50 mg acarbose and 41.7% with 100 mg acarbose and did not decrease significantly with voglibose (52).

Adverse effects are similar to those of other α-glucosidase inhibitors. The more common adverse effects are flatulence, diarrhea, and abdominal discomfort. Other adverse effects include dizziness and hypoglycemia (44).

Zenarestat

Zenarestat (Warner-Lambert) is in phase III development for the treatment of diabetic neuropathy. Zenarestat is an aldose reductase inhibitor. Aldose reductase inhibitors improve nerve conduction velocity and nerve morphology in diabetic peripheral polyneuropathy.

A randomized, placebo-controlled, double-blinded, multiple-dose, clinical trial with zenarestat was conducted over 52 weeks in patients with mild to moderate diabetic peripheral polyneuropathy. Zenarestat produced a dose-dependent effect on the sural nerve conduction velocity and decreased the sorbitol levels. The zenarestat doses that reduced sorbitol levels >80% were associated with an increase in the density of small-diameter (<5 μm) sural nerve myelinated fibers (53).

Zopolrestat

Preliminary reports indicate that zopolrestat (Alond; Pfizer) does not improve nerve function in patients with diabetic peripheral neuropathy. Development of this compound for the treatment of peripheral neuropathy has been suspended. However, it is still in phase II development for the treatment of diabetic nephropathy and cardiomyopathy (54).

REFERENCES

1. New Medicines in Development Database: Diabetes [online database]. Pharmaceutical Research and Manufacturers of America. Available at http://www.phrma.org/. Accessed 4 October 1999.

2. Schuster J, Rubsamen R, Lloyd P, Lloyd J: The AERx aerosol delivery system. *Pharm Res* 14:354–347, 1997

3. Kolterman O, Young G, Parker J, Amin D, Prickett K: Stimulation of endogenous insulin secretion by subcutaneous AC2993 (synthetic Exendin-4) in healthy overnight fasted volunteers (Abstract). *Diabetes* 48 (Suppl. 1):A199, 1999

4. Kiel D, Lakis JN, May JM: Exendin (9-39) is a partial agonist at the human glucagon-like peptide-1 receptor (Abstract). *Diabetes* 48 (Suppl. 1):A20, 1999

5. Salisbury L: New powder may break needle barrier for diabetics [online article]. *Reuters Health* 19 August 1999. Available at http://www.reutershealth.com. Accessed 19 August 1999.

6. Heinemann L, Heise T, Jorgensen LN, Starke AA: Action profile of the rapid acting insulin analogue: human insulin B28Asp. *Diabetic Med* 10:535–539, 1993

7. Heinemann L, Kapitza C, Starke AA, Heise T: Time-action profile of the insulin analogue B28Asp (Letter). *Diabetic Med* 13:683–687, 1996

8. Heinemann L, Weyer C, Rauhaus M, Heinrichs S, Heise T: Variability of the metabolic effect of soluble insulin and the rapid-acting insulin analog insulin aspart. *Diabetes Care* 21:1910–1914, 1998

9. Home PD, Lindholm A, Hylleberg B, Round P: Improved glycemic control with insulin aspart: a multicenter randomized double-blind crossover trial in type 1 diabetic patients. *Diabetes Care* 21:1904–1909, 1998

10. Lindholm A, McEwen J, Riis AP: Improved postprandial glycemic control with insulin aspart: a randomized double-blind cross-over trial in type 1 diabetes. *Diabetes Care* 22:801–805, 1998

11. Brange J, Volund A: Insulin analogs with improved pharmacokinetic profiles. *Adv Drug Delivery Rev* 35:307–335, 1999

12. Weyer C, Heise T, Heinemann L: Insulin aspart in a 30/70 premixed formulation: pharmacodynamic properties of a rapid-acting insulin analog in stable mixture. *Diabetes Care* 20:1612–1614, 1997

13. Wiefels K, Hubinger A, Dannehl K, Gries FA: Insulinkinetic and -dynamic in diabetic patients under insulin pump therapy after injections of human insulin or the insulin analogue (B28Asp). *Horm Metab Res* 27:421–424, 1995

14. Mudaliar SR, Lindberg FA, Joyce M, Beerdsen P, Strange P, Lin A, Henry RR: Insulin aspart (B28 asp-insulin): a fast-acting analog of human insulin: absorption kinetics and action profile compared with regular human insulin in healthy nondiabetic subjects. *Diabetes Care* 22:1501–1506, 1999

15. Humalog (lispro insulin) package insert, Eli Lilly, 1998

16. Rosskamp RH, Park G: Long-acting insulin analogs. *Diabetes Care* 22 (Suppl. 2):B109–B113, 1999

17. Berti L, Kellerer M, Bossenmaier B, Seffer E, Seipka G, Haring HU: The long acting human insulin analog HOE 901: characteristics of insulin signaling in comparison to Asp(B10) and regular insulin. *Horm Metab Res* 30:123–129, 1998

18. Liu L, Koenen M, Seipke G, Eckel J: IGF-I receptor-mediated signaling of the human insulin analogue HOE 901 (Abstract). *Diabetologia* 40 (Suppl. 1):A355, 1997

19. Bahr M, Kolter T, Seipke G, Eckel J: Growth promoting and metabolic activity of the human insulin analogue [Gly^{A21},Arg^{B31},Arg^{B32}]insulin (HOE 901) in muscle cells. *Eur J Pharmacol* 320:259–265, 1997

20. Tucker M: Recombinant product hailed as improvement over other insulins. *Biotechnology Newswatch*, 19 July 1999

21. Kramer W: New approaches to the treatment of diabetes. *Exp Clin Endocrinol* 107 (Suppl. 2):S52–S61, 1999

22. Lepore M, Kurzhals R, Pampanelli S, Fanelli CG, Bolli GB: Pharmacokinetics and dynamics of s.c. injection of the long-acting insulin glargine (HOE1) in T1DM (Abstract). *Diabetes* 48 (Suppl. 1):A97, 1999

23. Soon PC, Matthews DR, Rosskamp R, Herz M, Kurzhals R: 24 h profile of action of biosynthetic long-acting insulin (HOE901) tested in normal volunteers by glucose clamp methodology (Abstract). *Diabetes* 48 (Suppl. 1):A161, 1999

24. Linkeschowa R, Heise T, Rave K, Hompesch B, Sedlack M, Heinemann L: Time-action profile of the long-acting insulin analogue HOE901 (Abstract). *Diabetes* 48 (Suppl. 1):A97, 1999

25. Owens D, Luzio S, Beck P, Coates P, Tinbergen J, Kurzhals R: The absorption of the insulin analogue HOE 901 from different sites in healthy subjects (Abstract). *Diabetes* 46 (Suppl. 1):A329, 1997

26. Luzio SD, Owens D, Evans M, Ogunka A, Beck P, Kurzhals R: Comparison of the sc absorption of HOE 901 and NPH human insulin type 2 diabetic subjects (Abstract). *Diabetes* 48 (Suppl. 1):A111, 1999

27. Ratner RE, Hirsch I, Mecca T, Wilson C:: Efficacy and safety of insulin glargine in subjects with type 1 diabetes: a 28 week randomized, NPH insulin-controlled trial (Abstract). *Diabetes* 48 (Suppl. 1):A120, 1999

28. Witthaus E, Bradley C, Stewart J: Treatment satisfaction and psychological well-being in patients with type 1 diabetes, treated with a new long-acting insulin glargine (Abstract). *Diabetes* 48 (Suppl. 1):A353, 1999

29. Rosenstock J, Park G, Zimmerman J: Efficacy and safety of HOE 901 in patients with type 1 DM: a four-week randomized, NPH insulin-controlled trial (Abstract). *Diabetes* 47 (Suppl. 1):A92, 1998

30. Pieber TR, Eugene-Jolchine I, Derobert E, the European Study Group of HOE 901 in Type 1 Diabetes: Efficacy and safety of HOE 901 versus NPH insulin in patients with type 1 diabetes. *Diabetes Care* 23:157–162, 2000

31. Garg S, Gerard L, Pennington M, Mecca T, Taylor L, Chase P, Jennings K: Efficacy of the new long acting insulin analog (HOE901) on fasting glucose values in IDDM (Abstract). *Diabetes* 47 (Suppl. 1):A359, 1998

32. Rosenstock J, Schwartz S, Clark C, Edwards M, Donley D: Efficacy and safety of HOE 901 (insulin glargine) in subjects with type 2 DM:

a 28-week randomized, NPH insulin-controlled trial (Abstract). *Diabetes* 48 (Suppl. 1):A100, 1999

33. Raskin P, Park G, Zimmerman J: The effect of HOE 901 on glycemic control in type 2 diabetes (Abstract). *Diabetes* 47 (Suppl. 1):A103, 1998

34. Matthews DR, Pfeiffer C: Comparative clinical trial of a new long-acting insulin (HOE901) vs. protamine insulin demonstrates less nocturnal hypoglycaemia (Abstract). *Diabetes* 47 (Suppl. 1):A101, 1998

35. Hanefeld M, Bouter KP, Dickinson S, Guitard C: Rapid and short-acting mealtime insulin secretion with nateglinide controls both prandial and mean glycemia. *Diabetes Care* 23:202–207, 2000

36. De Souza C, Gagen K, Chen W, Dragonas N: Superior glycemic control with early insulin release versus total insulin release in type-2 diabetic rodent models (Abstract). *Diabetes* 48 (Suppl. 1):A270, 1999

37. Dunning BE, Gutierrez C: Pharmacodynamics of nateglinide and repaglinide in cynomolgus monkeys (Abstract). *Diabetes* 48 (Suppl. 1):A104, 1999

38. Dunning BE, Paladini S: Mimicking cephalic insulin release with the rapid-onset/short-duration insulinotrophic agent, nateglinide, reduces prandial glucose excursions without increasing total insulin exposure in IGT monkeys (Abstract). *Diabetes* 48 (Suppl. 1):A282, 1999

39. Hirschberg Y, McLeod J, Garreffa S, Spratt D: Pharmacodynamics and dose response of nateglinide type 2 diabetics (Abstract). *Diabetes* 48 (Suppl. 1):A100, 1999

40. Hirschberg Y, McLeod J, Garreffa S, Spratt D: Pharmacodynamics of nateglinide and dose response in patients with type 2 diabetes mellitus (Abstract). *Diabetes* 48 (Suppl. 1):A100, 1999

41. Kalbag J, Hirschberg Y, McLeod J, Garreffa S, Lasseter K: Comparison of mealtime glucose regulation by nateglinide and repaglinide in healthy subjects (Abstract). *Diabetes* 48 (Suppl. 1):A106, 1999

42. McLeod J, Hirschberg Y, Garreffa S, Keilson L, Mather S: Nateglinide enhances the physiological insulin response to a meal in type 2 diabetics (Abstract). *Diabetologia* 42 (Suppl. 1):A241, 1999

43. Friedman EA: Advanced glycosylated end products and hyperglycemia in the pathogenesis of diabetic complications. *Diabetes Care* 22 (Suppl. 2):B65–B71, 1999

44. Gelman CR, Rumack BH, Sayre NK (Eds.): *DRUGDEX System.* Vol 103; Edition expires 2/28/2000. Englewood, CO, MICROMEDEX

45. Amylin Pharmaceuticals reports positive results for Symlin in US Type 2 diabetes study [online article]. *PRNewswire*, 31 August 1999. Available at http://www.prnewswire.com. Accessed 31 August 1999.

46. Nyholm B, Orskov L, Hove KY, Gravholt CH, Moller N, Alberti KG, Moyses C, Kolterman O, Schmitz O: The amylin analog pramlintide improves glycemic control and reduces postprandial glucagon concentrations in patients with type 1 diabetes mellitus. *Metabolism* 48:935–941, 1999

47. Thompson RG, Pearson L, Schoenfeld SL, Kolterman OG: Pramlintide, a synthetic analog of human amylin, improves the metabolic profile of patients with type 2 diabetes using insulin: the Pramlintide in Type 2 Diabetes Group. *Diabetes Care* 21:987–993, 1998

48. Fineman M, Bahner A, Gottlieb A, Kolterman OG: Effects of six months administration of pramlintide as an adjunct to insulin therapy on metabolic control in people with type 1 diabetes (Abstract). *Diabetes* 48 (Suppl. 1):A113, 1999

49. Kolterman O, Bahner A, Gottlieb A, Fineman M: Pramlintide (human amylin analogue) as an adjunct to insulin therapy in patients with type 1 diabetes improved glycemic control over 2 years (Abstract). *Diabetes* 48 (Suppl. 1):A104, 1999

50. Hiraiwa M, Campana WM, Mizisin AP, Mohiuddin L, O'Brien JS: Prosaposin: a myelinotrophic protein that promotes expression of myelin constituents and is secreted after nerve injury. *Glia* 26:353–360, 1999

51. Matsumoto K, Yano M, Miyake S, Ueki Y, Yamaguchi Y, Akazawa S, Tominaga Y: Effects of voglibose on glycemic excursions, insulin secretion, and insulin sensitivity in non-insulin-treated type 2 diabetes patients. *Diabetes Care* 21:256–260, 1998

52. Kageyama S, Nakamichi N, Sekino H, Nakano S: Comparison of the effects of acarbose and voglibose in healthy subjects. *Clin Ther* 19:720–729, 1997

53. Greene DA, Arezzo JC, Brown MB: Effect of aldose reductase inhibition on nerve conduction and morphometry in diabetic neuropathy: Zenarestat Study Group. *Neurology* 53:580–591, 1999

54. Pfizer discontinues development of zopolrestat for diabetes indication [online article]. *Reuters Health*, 16 August 1999. Available at http://www.reutershealth.com. Accessed 16 August 1999

55. Toft-Nielsen MB, Madsbad S, Holst JJ: Continuous subcutaneous infusion of glucagon-like peptide 1 lowers plasma glucose and reduces appetite in type 2 diabetic patients. *Diabetes Care* 22:1137–1143, 1999

56. Mizuno K, Kato N, Makino M, Suzuki T, Shindo M: Continuous inhibition of excessive polyol pathway flux in peripheral nerves by aldose reductase inhibitor fidarestat leads to improvement of diabetic neuropathy. *J Diabetes Complications* 13:141–150, 1999

57. Herz M: Clinical update on Humalog® Mix25™ a novel pre-mixed formulation of insulin lispro and NPL. *IJCP* 104 (Suppl.):8–13, 1999

58. Treating diabetes: Desmos and TheraCyte to test combined technologies [online article]. *PRNewswire*, 16 August 1999. Available at http://www.prnewswire.com. Accessed 16 August 1999

59. Bristol-Myers Squibb files new drug application for novel oral antidiabetic drug [online article]. *PRNewswire*, 30 September 1999. Available at http://www.prnewswire.com. Accessed 30 September 1999.

60. EASD: Researchers report enhanced insulin response with exendin-4 in type 2 diabetes [online article]. *Doctor's Guide to Medical & Other News*, 30 September 1999. Available at http://www.pslgroup.com. Accessed 30 September 1999.

61. Anon.: NovoNordisk close to US FDA approval for fast-acting insulin. *Bloomberg News*, 17 September 1999. Available at AOL Bloomberg News. Accessed 17 September 1999.

62. Leslie CA: New insulin replacement technologies: overcoming barriers to tight glycemic control. *Clev Clin J Med* 66:293–302, 1999

63. Reents S, Seymour J (Ed.): *Clin Pharmacology*. Gold Standard Multimedia, 1999. Available at http://www.gsm.com. Accessed 3 September 1999.

64. Andreis PG, Malendowicz LK, Neri G, Tortorella C, Nussdorfer GG: Effects of glucagon and glucagon-like peptide-1 on glucocorticoid secretion of dispersed rat adrenocortical cells. *Life Sci* 64:2187–2197, 1999

65. Sprague KL (Ed.): Formulary's Resource Guide to Pharmaceutical Manufacturers. *Formulary* (Suppl.):1–110, 1999

Index